MW01231907

THE ULTIMATE

GASTRIC SLEEVE

BARIATRIC

COOKBOOK

Delicious Recipes to Enjoy Your Favorite Foods for a Sustainable Weight Loss and a Healthy Life.

SUMMER KELLY

TABLE OF CONTENTS

ABOUT GASTRIC SLEEVE SURGERY

WHAT IS GASTRIC SLEEVE SURGERY

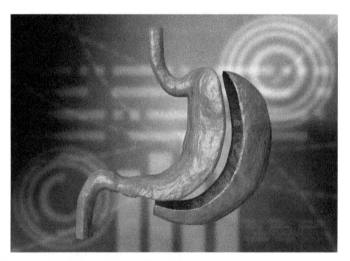

Diagram: Post Gastric Sleeve Surgery Stomach

Vertical sleeve gastrectomy, also known as gastric sleeve surgery, is a process in which the stomach's capacity to hold the food is reduced by 80 percent. In other words, a sleeve is created on the side of the stomach, which receives the food in a small amount; the rest is separated through this surgery.

This bariatric procedure is also called weight loss surgery as it is used to induce weight loss through a permanent approach. The diagram shows how the stomach walls are stitched together to create a separate sleeve for food digestion.

WHY IS IT NEEDED?

The gastric sleeve surgery is mainly opted to achieve weight loss. This surgery works for people who are sensitive to dietary changes and just can't lose weight through diet control. So, this surgery finds a permanent solution and reduces the stomach size, which automatically cuts down food consumption.

This surgery has given effective results, and within one year of the surgery, people should 70 percent weight loss. By controlling obesity, such individuals were also able to resist diabetes, insulin resistance, sleep apnea, hypertension, joints pain, fatty liver disease, and hyperlipidemia. Excessive hunger sensation is also reduced to a minimum after gastric sleeve surgery.

The procedure is indeed effective, but it works well only when a person changes his dietary habits after the surgery and follows a gastric sleeve diet.

Pre-Surgery Tips:

- Change your diet and switch to a liquid-only diet a week before the surgery.
- If you are a smoker, then stop smoking at least 2 weeks before the surgery to avoid complications.

- Discuss your health condition and post-surgery effects with your doctor before the surgery.
- Clean your kitchen and set up the pantry according to the new lifestyle.
- Increase the protein intake to prepare the body for quick recovery after the surgery.

Post-Surgery Tips

- Switch to the gastric sleeve diet and use more clear liquids right after the surgery.
- Add protein-based supplements and liquids to the diet to ensure quick recovery and healing of the stomach.
- Start with the intake of soft food and gradually switch to the proper meals.
- Stop having heavy, oily food on the table.
- Light exercises and yoga ensure quick recovery, so try some light exercises 2-3 days after the surgery.
- Consult your dietician and the doctor after every week to discuss your diet and changing health conditions.

GASTRIC SLEEVE DIET

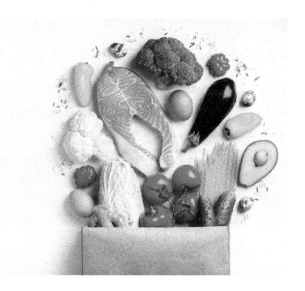

WHAT IS A GASTRIC SLEEVE DIET?

Gastric diet is one of the strict diet plans followed before and after gastric sleeve surgery. It strictly reduces the intake of calories and carbohydrates. These calories and carbohydrates are coming from sweets, pasta, and potatoes. During gastric sleeve diet, you have to consume liquid foods that are low in calories and high in protein. Protein helps to maintain your muscle mass and also helps to maintain your body energy level.

Before two days of surgery, you have to switch to a clear liquid diet, such as sugar-free protein shake, decaffeinated coffee or tea, sugar-free popsicles, broth, and water. During the gastric sleeve diet, completely avoid caffeinated and carbonated beverages. After gastric sleeve surgery, a person must follow a strict diet to recover your body and adjust to the smaller size of your stomach. The person with gastric sleeve surgery eats smaller and more frequent meals for the rest of their lives. The diet plan can be divided into four stages:

STAGE ONE DIET: CLEAR LIQUIDS

This stage is beginning in the first week after your gastric sleeve surgery. In this stage of the diet, only a few ounces of food drinks have been allowed. This will help your stomach heal without getting stretched by foods. The liquid diet includes:

- Water
- Thin soup and broth
- Skim milk
- Decaffeinated coffee and tea
- Sugar-free gelatin and popsicles
- Unsweetened juice.

Avoid sugary liquids during the first week of gastric sleeve surgery. Consuming sugary drinks may lead to raising digestive problems and occurs negative side effect on surgery. Also, avoid carbonated and caffeinated beverages. During the first week of surgery, always stay your body hydrated, just remember only drink a small amount of liquid at a time.

STAGE TWO DIET: PROTEIN-RICH LIQUIDS

The stage two begins after five days of gastric sleeve surgery. During this stage, you have to allow consuming protein-rich shake and more liquids like Skimmed milk, unsweetened, and blended fruit juice. During this stage, you experience an increase in your appetite, but you have to stick to your diet plan for getting a positive result.

The protein-rich liquid includes:

- Sugar-free protein shakes
- Thin creamed soup and broth
- Non-fat sugar-free puddings
- Low-carb yogurt
- Split pea or lentil soup
- All food in stage one.

During stage two it recommends you to consume about 3 liters of liquid diet per day. Avoid sugary and carbonated liquids during stage two.

STAGE THREE DIET: PUREE

Stage three begins after two weeks of gastric sleeve surgery. It allows you to include pureed soft food into your diet. The foods like mashed potatoes, fat-free yogurts, thick and smooth soups, baked beans. You are allowed to eat these diets in small quantity about 4 to 5 times daily.

Food allowed during stage three is:

- Puree no sugar added fruits
- Tofu
- Pureed peas and lentils
- Eggs

- Plain yogurt
- Steamed or boiled vegetables.

STAGE FOUR DIET: SOLID FOOD

Stage four begins after the four weeks of gastric sleeve surgery. It allows you to take soft solid food in the diet. Try to consume protein-rich foods because it recommends that you should consume at least 60 grams of protein in your daily meal.

At this stage, your stomach should be fit to handle solid food. During this stage, you can consume three meals with some snacks. The solid foods allowed in this stage are:

- Lentil and beans soup
- Hot cereals
- Fish
- Boil potatoes
- Soft fruits without skin
- Low-fat cheese
- Lean ground turkey, chicken, beef, pork
- Cooked vegetables.

During this stage, you should avoid whole milk products, snacks, and sugary drinks, fibrous vegetables like broccoli, celery, asparagus, starchy foods like white potatoes, pasta and bread, spicy foods, processed and fried fast food, ETC.

HOW DOES THE GASTRIC SLEEVE WORK?

After gastric sleeve surgery, your stomach is holding a smaller amount of food because during surgery near about 75 to 80 percent of parts of your stomach are removed from your body. It helps you to reduce your food carving and weight loss process.

The surgery also removes the part of the stomach that produces Ghrelin. Ghrelin is one of the gut hormones produced in your stomach, it is also called hunger hormones. Removing these hormones from your body will reduce your hunger feeling and also help to reduce your appetite. By removing these hormones from your stomach, you can easily reduce you're overweight.

ADVANTAGES OF SURGERY

Gastric Bariatric Sleeve Surgery is an insignificantly obtrusive medical procedure to decrease the size of the stomach. It is currently the most mainstream weight reduction in medical procedures all around the world. People frequently observe the extraordinary achievement that their loved ones have had with the sleeve surgery and, at that point, need similar outcomes.

Patients accomplish substantial weight reduction with a straightforward activity without too much stress. It bodes well that with a little stomach, you will be able to eat less and lose a lot of weight. The sleeve surgery has been seen as substantially more potent than the gastric band surgery. It does not require the arrangement of an outside gadget or needle modifications, which the later needs.

Following are some advantages that come alongside this surgery:

Hauling around unreasonable weight puts a great deal of pressure on your joints, regularly causing incessant agony and joint harm. The noteworthy and supported weight reduction that happens after bariatric medical procedures diminishes the weight on joints and regularly permits individuals to quit utilizing torment prescriptions and appreciate considerably more mobility.

Accomplishing and supporting a typical weight territory regularly permits individuals with rest apnea to quit utilizing a CPAP machine at sleep time.

Bariatric medical procedure causes long haul reduction of hard-to-control type 2 diabetes. The aftereffects of this strategy are exceptionally viable for obese or overweight patients with type 2 diabetes, permitting practically all patients to stay liberated from insulin and subordinate prescriptions for about three years post the medical procedure.

Numerous hefty individuals feel discouraged due to helpless self-perception and social shame. Considerably more young individuals who convey a critical abundance of weight think that it is hard to partake in exercises they may somehow appreciate, prompting social separation and discouragement that lead to depression. Losing this weight can enhance enthusiastic well-being in these patients.

Weight reduction medical procedure can likewise improve fertility conditions during childbearing years.

Weight reduction medical procedure can mitigate metabolic disorder, pregnancy entanglements, gallbladder ailment, and that is just the beginning.

With heftiness and its related wellbeing inconveniences increasing at an alarming rate in the world, bariatric medical procedure unquestionably speaks to be an incredible asset for giving supported alleviation to overweight individuals.

LIFE POST-BARIATRIC SURGERY

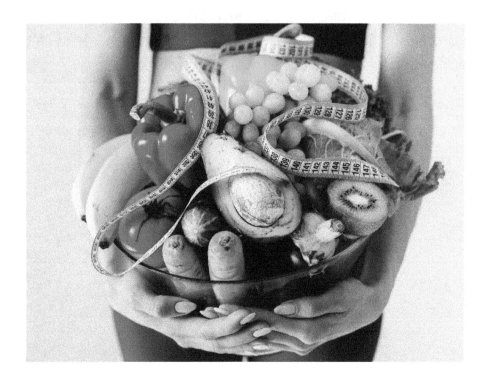

STAGE ONE

Food and Drink Choices

You need to follow your doctor's orders as far as when, how much, and what foods you can consume after your gastric sleeve surgery. However, this guide can give you an idea of what to expect.

Surgery day - The staff will put you on intravenous fluid, but you will have to drink about one fluid ounce of water (and only water) per hour. You will be given one-ounce medicine cups to measure out and sip your water from, and you will be required to make notes regarding your water intake.

Day One - Usually by noon on the day following your surgery, you will start to consume between one and three ounces of broth, sugar-free gelatin, decarbonized ("flat") diet ginger ale, or water per hour.

You will need to stop drinking as soon as you feel full. Don't force yourself to drink more than you are comfortable drinking. However, the goal will be for you to reach a drinking capacity of one quart (32 ounces) per day. You will likely reach that goal within that day. Once you do, the intravenous fluids can be discontinued.

Day Two - Usually by the second day out from your surgery, you will take in low-sugar, enriched liquids. You will do this for two to three weeks.

You will take in four fluid ounces of a nutritional supplement every other hour over an eight-hour period per day. Between these supplements, you will drink between four and eight fluid ounces of various clear liquids. These liquids include the following:

- Decaffeinated herbal tea
- Decaffeinated coffee
- Fruit juice (no added sugar, max 4 ounces per serving and 8 ounces daily)
- Sugar-free popsicles (under 20 calories, up to two daily)
- Tomato juice
- V-8 juice
- Flat diet decaffeinated soda
- Broth
- Sugar-free drinks like kool-aid or crystal light
- Water.

Fluid goal: The fluid goal is for you to reach a capacity of six cups of liquid per day of both the nutrient-enriched beverage and the clear liquids. Stop when full, though, and don't push things beyond what is comfortable.

Protein goal: You will need to consume at least 70 grams of protein per day, which is usually what is in seven scoops of protein powder. You will need to track your protein intake.

Supplements: Take these with your meals. You will need to take two multivitamins in chewable form in addition to three 600 mg of calcium carbonate and vitamin D in chewable form daily.

Reminders: Take 30 minutes to sip your liquids and continue to record all food and fluid intake.

The Clear Liquids Diet

A clear liquid diet is recommended in the post-op stage after the gastric sleeve surgery. It is mainly because that few days after the surgery, the healing phase initiates, and the stomach isn't capable of processing nutrients and calories in the food, but the body does need hydration. Clear liquid provides much-needed minerals, metabolites, and moisture that the body needs; therefore, they are given to a person after the surgery for a quick recovery. The following are the clear liquids that must be consumed on the bariatric diet.

- Broth
- Unsweetened juice
- Decaffeinated tea or coffee
- Milk (skim or 1 percent)
- Sugar-free gelatine drinks.

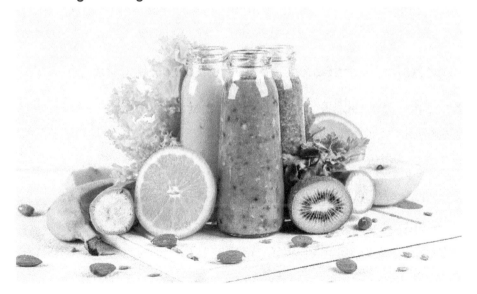

The rule of thumb for clear liquids is that it's either you can see through the glass—side to side or the water is thin enough that it's flowing freely, and you can somehow see through from side to side. You are to consume only light liquids for the following 2 to 3 days or after your admission from the hospital.

Examples of clear liquids you can consume after the surgery include:

- Tap water
- Pure fruit juices – refrain from drinking commercially processed or powdered juices.
- Broths or soups– vegetables, beef, or chicken are okay, but make sure that it's clear and no solid sediments are present.
- Other clear liquids may include decaffeinated coffee or tea and calorie-free sports drink.

Important Notes Before You Delve into These Recipes

Keeping yourself hydrated is the most crucial part a few days after your surgery. You should drink 48 to 64 ounces or 6 to 8 glass of water per day.

Never serve recipes either cold or hot for around 6 weeks until you have fully recovered from the surgery. Consuming extreme foods might cause gastric problems and compromise surgical procedure.

When consuming fruit juices, make sure that they are fresh

and natural. Also, dilute them thoroughly to obtain a steady liquid consistency and strain them to remove excess solid compounds. This process is to avoid the development of diarrhea or nausea.

However, you have to bear in mind that your stomach is still recovering after surgery. Thus, you may still experience episodes of nausea or vomiting, but these are common, and you have nothing to worry about. Again, we emphasize that you always hydrate yourself to alleviate the above symptoms.

Also, it has to be noted that food choices during this phase are limited. Thus, the recipes presented below are easy and simple to make, which mainly revolves around broths and juices.

Also, you don't really have to concern yourself with what to prepare because the hospital got you covered. They will provide the necessary clear liquids to aid your recovery process. But if you want to add a personal touch to your meals, then the following recipes are guaranteed delicious and, most importantly, nutritious and aid recovery.

Pure Fruit Juices: Important reminder: since solid compounds are not allowed for a few days after surgery, you have to take extra precautionary steps. While blenders liquefy solid foods, some solid compounds may still peak through. Thus, we recommend you to use strainers in each of the juice recipes to remove solid compounds.

GOOD CHOICES OF CLEAR FLUIDS

1. Water.

2. Tea – warm traditional, fruit or herbal teas.
3. Coffee – warm, ideally decaffeinated.
4. 'No-added-sugar' or 'sugar-free' squashes and cordials.
5. Bovril, marmite or oxo 'salty' drinks diluted well with hot water.
6. Sugar-free ice lollies.
7. Sugar-free jelly, made up as per packet instructions.
8. Chicken, beef or vegetable bouillon/broth/consommé or clear soup.
9. A whey protein isolate fruit drink like syntrax nectar, made up with water –great for getting protein in the early days.

ASIAN PEAR/BEET JUICE

| 5 min | 0 min | Liquids Diet | 2 Servings |

INGREDIENTS

- 1 Asian pear
- 1 apple
- 1 beet
- 1 carrot
- ½ cup cabbage
- 3 handfuls chard.

DIRECTIONS

1. Juice all the ingredients in the order listed according to the manufacturer's instructions.

1. Serve immediately.

NUTRITION (per serving):

Calories: 123 kcal | Fats: 0g | Carbs: 19g | Protein: 1g.

FRESH GREEN JUICE

5 min

0 min

Liquids Diet

2 Servings

INGREDIENTS

- 5-6 kale leaves
- 1 cucumber
- 3-4 celery stalks
- 2 apples
- ½ lemon, peeled or sliced.

DIRECTIONS

1. Juice all the ingredients in the order listed according to the manufacturer's instructions.

2. Serve immediately.

NUTRITION (per serving):

Calories: 53 kcal | Fats: 0g | Carbs: 13g | Protein: 1g.

CARROT PINEAPPLE ORANGE JUICE

5 min

0 min

Liquids Diet

2 Servings

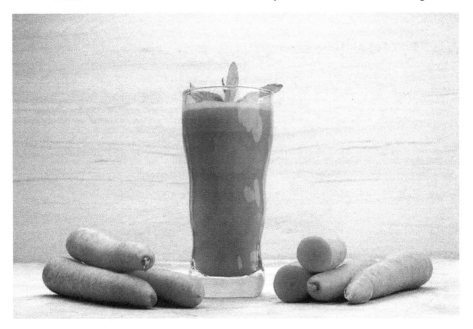

INGREDIENTS

- 1 small orange, including rind, seeded and cut into pieces
- ⅛ small, ripe pineapple, peeled, cored and cut into

DIRECTIONS

1. Juice all the ingredients in the order listed according to the manufacturer's instructions.

2. Serve immediately.

pieces

- 2 carrots, scrubbed clean and cut into pieces

- ½ lemon juice, stirred in at end.

NUTRITION (per serving):

Calories: 113 kcal | Fats: 0g | Carbs: 9g | Protein: 0g.

RICH ANTIOXIDANT JUICE

| 5 min | 0 min | Liquids Diet | 2 Servings |

INGREDIENTS

- 3 medium carrots, peeled
- 2 medium beets, cleaned and brushed
- 1 Green apple such as Granny Smith, peeled and cored.

DIRECTIONS

1. Juice all the ingredients in the order listed according to the manufacturer's instructions.

2. Serve immediately.

NUTRITION (per serving):

Calories: 123 kcal | Fats: 0g | Carbs: 19g | Protein: 1g.

BLOOD ORANGE SPORTS DRINK

5 min

0 min

Liquids Diet

2 Servings

INGREDIENTS

- 2 cups of coconut water
- 1 medium blood orange, squeezed
- 1½ tbsp. of honey or 1 packet of Stevia sugar
- Pinch of salt.

DIRECTIONS

1. Combine all ingredients together and mix well.
2. Serve immediately.

NUTRITION (per serving):

Calories: 234 kcal | Fats: 4g | Carbs: 27g | Protein: 2g.

LIME & MINT INFUSION

5 min

0 min

Liquids Diet

2 Servings

INGREDIENTS

- 2 cups of cold water
- 1 large lime, sliced
- ½ cup of lightly packed spearmint leaves
- 1 package of Stevia sugar.

DIRECTIONS

1. In a 1-quart glass container or larger, lightly mash the lime and spearmint leaves with the pestle.

2. Add iced cold water. Stir well.

3. Optional: add Stevia to taste.

NUTRITION (per serving):

Calories: 75 kcal | Fats: 0g | Carbs: 23g | Protein: 0g.

STRAWBERRY ICED TEA

5 min

0 min

Liquids Diet

2 Servings

INGREDIENTS

- 6-10 medium strawberries, chopped
- 1 tsp. lemon juice
- 2 cups of brewed white tea, chilled
- ½ - 1 tsp. honey or Stevia sugar (optional).

DIRECTIONS

1. Puree the strawberries until smooth consistency. Then strain through fine cheesecloth on top of a metal strainer to remove the seeds.

2. Combine the strained strawberry mixture with lemon juice and white tea.

3. Mix well. Add honey or Stevia to taste.

NUTRITION (per serving):

Calories: 127 kcal | Fats: 0g | Carbs: 24g | Protein: 1g.

WATERMELON POPSICLES

5 min

0 min

Liquids Diet

2 Servings

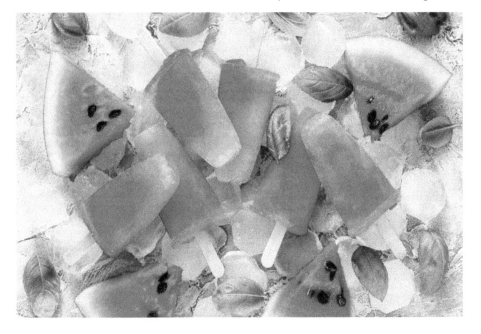

INGREDIENTS

- 2 cups watermelon juice (no sugar added store bought juice or homemade freshly pressed juice)
- ½ tbsp. lime juice
- 1 tsp. honey or

DIRECTIONS

1. Mix all ingredients together.
2. Carefully transfer mixture to the mold of your choice.
3. Freeze overnight.

Stevia sugar
(optional).

NUTRITION (per serving):

Calories: 135 kcal | Fats: 0g | Carbs: 22g | Protein: 1g.

HOMEMADE CHICKEN BROTH

15 min

2 h 30 min

Liquids Diet

6 Servings

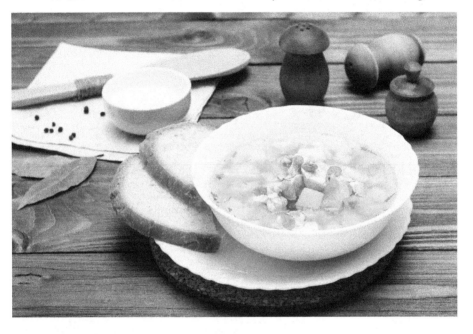

INGREDIENTS

- 2 lbs. bone-in skin on chicken
- 2 large carrots, cleaned and thick sliced
- 2 medium onions, quartered
- 3 celery sticks with

DIRECTIONS

1. Combine everything in a pot except the salt. Bring to a boil.

2. Skim the floating foam.

3. Lower the heat. Simmer for about 2 hours until the meat can be easily removed from the bone.

4. Strain vegetables, bones, meats, and spices from the broth and

leaves, cut into
chunks

- 8 whole
peppercorns

- 1 tsp. thyme, dried

- 1 tsp. rosemary,
dried

- 2 cups of water

- Salt to taste.

discard the solids.

5. Season broth with salt to taste.

6. Let the broth cool or refrigerate overnight. Skim the fat for a leaner broth.

NUTRITION (per serving):

Calories: 75 kcal | Fats: 0g | Carbs: 23g | Protein: 0g.

GINGER CHICKEN SOUP

| 15 min | 2 h 30 min | Liquids Diet | 6 Servings |

Healthy and lean homemade chicken soup with garlic, ginger, and lemongrass. The aromatic lemongrass add freshness to the broth with a hint of spiciness from the ginger. The best to enjoy this broth warm. This homemade chicken stock can be refrigerated for 2 days or frozen for 1 month to prolong shelf life.

INGREDIENTS

- 6-10 medium strawberries, chopped
- 1 tsp. lemon juice
- 2 cups of brewed white tea, chilled
- ½ - 1 tsp. honey or Stevia sugar (optional).

DIRECTIONS

1. Puree the strawberries until smooth consistency. Then strain through fine cheesecloth on top of a metal strainer to remove the seeds.

2. Combine the strained strawberry mixture with lemon juice and white tea.

3. Mix well. Add honey or Stevia to taste.

NUTRITION (per serving):

Calories: 127 kcal | Fats: 0g | Carbs: 24g | Protein: 1g.

POST OPERATION
SOFT & PUREED FOODS

STAGE TWO

Two to Three Weeks Out – Two or three weeks after your surgery, you can gradually introduce pureed and soft food that resembles the consistency of applesauce and up to a very soft consistency.

You will consume thick liquids, such as protein shakes and pureed food, using your blender for most of what you consume during this phase. Because of their high protein content, the protein shakes will be useful to you on days when you are having trouble reaching your daily intake of protein.

You won't be using a straw (because it might introduce air to your stomach), but the food will need to be blended so small that it could fit through a straw. Your pureed food will resemble baby food. In fact, you can eat baby food, but only the pureed meat ones contain the protein you need. You will probably enjoy pureed meat that you make yourself better, though.

You may not be able to tolerate meat until later on in this stage. You can see how you do with meat later on if you want to. There are many other tasty choices available that will give you the protein and other nutrients you need.

You need to have six meals per day and take the supplements and liquids in between meal times, not with the meals. Remember to chew well all food that needs to be chewed.

SOFT/PUREED FOOD COOKING TIPS AND MENU IDEAS FOR YOUR STAGE TWO DIET

You'll want to ease into this stage by consuming things like Lactaid-free milk, almond milk, unsweetened coconut milk, blended Greek yogurt with no fruit chunks, unsweetened applesauce, cooked cereal such as oatmeal, grits, or Cream of Wheat made with lactose-free milk, blended soup made with lactose-free milk, blended fruit smoothies, and shakes.

Do not combine food selections below right at first in any one meal, but gradually try the following foods during this phase:

- Light white fish
- Crackers with peanut butter
- Cooked eggs
- Cooked vegetables
- Soft fruit
- Yogurt with fruit
- Cottage cheese

- Oatmeal, grits, or Cream of Wheat
- Blended soup.

You may tolerate meat, however, so you can test your tolerance and see. After all, you won't want to only consume breakfast food and sweet-tasting shakes for longer than you have to. Below, you can find sources of protein and also food from the various food groups that you ought to begin to consume during this phase.

PROTEIN SOURCES

Protein is essential for our bodies to function properly, and you need to concentrate on consuming liquid protein when you first get out of your surgery. Protein will speed up the healing process, enhance your fat-burning metabolism, and minimize your hair loss.

Besides a deficiency in protein, hair loss is also associated with a deficiency in iron and zinc, so you'll need to make sure you take multivitamins. You will probably lose some hair anyway about a half year after your surgery for a little bit, so you will want to be sure that you give it all of the nutrients that you can to eventually come out of this experience thin, with muscle tone and a full head of hair.

Eat lots of protein and take your vitamins! You'll need to take in around 70 grams of protein per day during this phase. Remember that you will need to mash or puree foods that are not already soft. Here are some good sources of protein:

PROTEIN SOURCE	Serving Size	Gr. Per Serving
Protein powders (for smoothies)	1 scoop	20-40
Cooked vegetables	.5 cup	1-2
Instant breakfast drinks	1 packet	4-15
Tofu	3 oz.	11
Soy veggie burger	1	9
Bread	1 slice	2
Rice	.5 cup	5
Noodles/macaroni	.5 cup	3-4
Dry cereal	1 oz.	5
Oatmeal	1 cup	5
Nuts	.25 cup	4.5
Lima beans	.5 cup	5
Peanut butter	2 tbsp.	8.5
Beans: brown, kidney, black-eyed peas garbanzo, white, pinto, black	.5 cup	7.5
Fat-free refried beans	.5 cup	8
Reduced-fat ricotta cheese	1 oz.	6
Low-fat yogurt	1 cup	8-12
Non-fat milk powder	1 tbsp.	2.5
Skim milk/1% milk	1 cup	8
Low-fat cottage cheese	.5 cup	13
Egg substitute	.25 cup	6
Egg whites	2 tbsp.	9
Egg	1 med	7
Lean meat: pork, beef, fish, chicken	1 oz.	7

Other sources of protein include:

- Nonfat dry milk powder (Add this to hot cereals, soups, casseroles, etc.)
- Legumes

- Fish
- Cream of Wheat with skim milk
- Strained cream soups, such as chicken, mushroom, potato, or celery
- Baby food meats
- White fish, such as orange roughy, tilapia, haddock, and cod
- Canned chicken breast
- Canned tuna in water.

Grains and Starches

You will need to mash or puree foods that are not already soft. Good sources of grains and starches include the following:

- Winter squash
- Mashed potatoes
- Sweet potatoes
- Baby oatmeal
- Grits
- Farina.

Fruit

You will need to mash or puree foods that are not already soft. Good sources of fruit include the following:

- Peaches
- Apricots
- Melons
- Pineapples
- Pears

- Bananas
- Canned fruit in own juices
- Applesauce
- Juice sweetened with a non-nutritive sweetener
- Diluted 100% apple juice
- Diluted 100% grape juice
- Diluted 100% cranberry juice.

Vegetables

You will need to mash or puree foods that are not already soft. Good sources of vegetables include the following:

- Diet V-8 Splash
- V-8 Juice
- Other tomato juice
- Spinach
- Green beans
- Summer squash
- Carrots.

Note: Avoid cauliflower, broccoli, or other fibrous veggies during your stage two, pureed food time.

Drinks

Make sure that you consume at least eight cups of low-calorie, caffeine-free liquids throughout the day so that you will prevent yourself from becoming dehydrated. Sip these drinks between the meals. Do not drink with meals. Wait for 30 to 45 minutes after you finish your meal before you drink fluids. The following items are examples of drinks you can have:

- Sugar-free flavored drinks
- Skim milk
- Decaffeinated coffee (maximum 8 ounces per day)
- Decaffeinated tea (maximum 8 ounces per day)
- Diet fruit drinks (under 10 calories per day)
- Water
- Sugar-free flavored water
- Zero-calorie flavored water.

Supplements

You will also need to start taking supplements daily that contain the following:

- Iron
- Zinc
- Calcium citrate
- B12
- Other supplements as indicated from your lab results.

Take them in chewable form for the first month (something like Flintstones) twice daily. You can start taking vitamins and minerals in pill form after your first post-operative month if you prefer pills.

LACTOSE AND FOOD INTOLERANCES

Some gastric sleeve patients become intolerant to lactose after their surgery, so you'll need to use unsweetened coconut milk, almond milk, or Lactaid-free milk. If you have pain or vomit after you introduce a new kind of food, go back to your liquid diet for an entire day before trying pureed food again. Don't let it discourage you. Notate when you ate the problem food, what food it was that gave you the problem, and what your reaction was to it.

You may not be able to tolerate poultry or other meat for a while after your surgery. If you have trouble tolerating some of the pureed meat, you might want to wait until later in this phase to try meat. You can just label it and freeze it.

Alternatively, you can introduce meat in small amounts, blended in with potatoes or other vegetables and/or sauces. There are recipes for meat dishes in this book that you can make. Many of them are various veggie-rich meatball and sauce meals that you eat in blended form while you are in the early stages after your gastric sleeve surgery.

Food to Avoid

Sugar and carbs can easily sabotage your weight loss efforts, as can bad fats or even good fats if eaten excess. Avoid the following foods to prevent sabotaging your weight loss efforts:

- Fried food
- Doughnuts
- Alcohol
- Ice cream
- Sherbet
- Preserves
- Cakes
- Molasses
- Flavored drink mix

- Honey
- Regular sodas
- Sweets
- Candy.

TIPS FOR THE FIRST MONTH AFTER YOUR OPERATION

Keep food records. You may want to do this indefinitely, just to stay on top of what you're eating, but be sure to do it for that first after your surgery. Notate the following:

- Time you ate
- Type of food you ate
- Amount of food you ate
- How you prepared your food, including any oils used
- Protein gram amount wherever you can find this information.

Use ice trays to control portion size, noting that each cube holds about two ounces. These are good for use with pureed meats and vegetables, low-fat cream soups, etc.

Eat only two to four ounces of food per meal, concentrating on protein intake. Try to get 80 grams of protein daily, which protein shakes and supplements would help you to achieve in addition to what you can eat.

Try to eat between four and six small meals daily.

Take your time eating and drinking. Take half an hour to eat and drink just four ounces, which is half a cup.

Drink at least eight cups of liquids daily between the meals, waiting 30 to 45 minutes after your last meal to drink.

LOW-FAT COOKING TIPS

When you get to where you can eat more solid food, prepare the food items as normal and then just puree/blend or mash them. See how you like the taste. If you don't tolerate meat by itself, you may tolerate a little of it if it is mixed with mashed potatoes, along with low-fat sour cream, or eaten in blended recipe form (See the blended meat recipes).

Poultry and Other Meat

- Use lean meat.
- Top round beef (It's best to forego red meat, however)
- Turkey, no skin, white meat
- Chicken, no skin, white meat
- Trim off the fat
- Use low-fat cooking methods
- Broil, grill, bake, sauté, stir-fry using broth, vegetable spray, a small amount of oil, or water
- Drain off fat.

Vegetables

- Use "I Can't Believe It's Not Butter" spray for butter flavor without the calories.
- Add tomatoes, carrots, green peppers, and other fresh vegetables to your spaghetti sauces.
- Add fat-free sour cream or low-fat cottage cheese to potatoes.

- Cook using methods that do not require fat, such as microwave, steam, grill, and bake.
- Don't cook with bacon, butter, or fatback.
- Avoid high-fat sauces, such as butter, oil, cheese, and sauces made with cream.

Soups

- Let your soup cool. Skim fat off after it has cooled, accumulated on the top, and hardened.

Desserts

- Use Splenda to add sweetness to smoothies, shakes, unsweetened decaffeinated tea, etc.
- Read food labels. Only consider food items that have low sugar content or use artificial sweeteners.

Soft Foods

When you transitioned to phase 3 of your recovery process, you can now move on to more solid foods, which include whole-wheat cereals, fish, chicken, vegetables, and fresh fruits.

Things to keep in mind after the first month of recovery:

1. Chew your food thoroughly before swallowing.
2. Continue to drink your 6 to 8 cups of water.
3. Intake of high-protein foods or supplements. Consume them before meals. The General recommended intake is 50 to 60 grams of protein for women and 60 to 70 grams for men.
4. In consuming dietary supplements, choose those that are chewable.

5. Refrain from eating foods that contain high levels of calories.
6. Do not drink while you're eating. Doing so can cause your stomach to fill quickly.
7. Drink liquids 30 minutes after you've finished your meal.
8. Because you'll be restricting calorie intake, it's essential that you take dietary supplements regularly.

GOOD CHOICES OF FULL LIQUIDS

1. Milk – skimmed, semi-skimmed, almond, soya, oat, rice and Flora Proactive.
2. Milky chai type tea – lightly-spiced for added flavors.
3. Yogurt without added sugar and fruit bits.
4. Whey protein isolate drinks, icy, cold or warm made up with milk or water.
5. Ice cream made with whey protein isolate powder mixed with milk or water.
6. Mashed potato mixed with a little broth or gravy until thin and soup-like.
7. Fresh homemade fruit juice without added sugar and diluted with water.
8. V8 or tomato juice – warm or chilled.
9. Home-made, not too thick smoothies diluted if necessary, with water.
10. Simple home-made cocoa (made with 2 tablespoons unsweetened cocoa powder and 1 cup semi-skimmed milk).
11. Unsweetened and low-fat hot chocolate drinks.
12. Smooth cream-style low-fat soups.

13. Home-made vegetable, fish or poultry soups, pureed until smooth and diluted to a smooth runny consistency (gradually increase the thickness as you progress through this stage to the next soft or pureed food stage).
14. Very gently set egg custards.
15. Low-sugar and low-fat custards.

GOOD CHOICES OF SOFT FOODS

1. Porridge, oat with semi-skimmed milk and runny consistency.
2. Mashed banana with a little yogurt if liked or with a low-fat and low-sugar custard.
3. Scrambled eggs cooked very soft.
4. Very soft and gently cooked plain omelet.
5. A soft-boiled egg or poached one.
6. Plain low-fat cottage cheese.
7. Low-sugar and low-fat fromage frais.
8. Pureed chicken or turkey in gravy.
9. Pureed fish (salmon, tuna, pilchards or mackerel) in a thin tomato sauce.
10. Soft and smooth low-fat pate or spread.
11. Pureed boiled vegetables such as potato, pumpkin, cauliflower or carrot with thin gravy or mixed with grated low-fat cheese or low-fat cream cheese.
12. Pureed casserole and stew dishes of a thinnish consistency.
13. Pureed, thickened or soft piece vegetable and chicken soups.
14. Smooth and light low-sugar and low-fat milk mousse.

15. Milky pudding such as tapioca, sago or rice but keep sugar to a minimum.
16. Soft lentils, beans and peas, mashed or pureed for a little texture.
17. Silken or smooth tofu.
18. Thick fruit and vegetable smoothies.
19. Pureed avocado.
20. Low-sugar sorbets.

GREEN BOOSTER SMOOTHIE

 5 min

 0 min

 Soft &Pureed food

 2 Servings

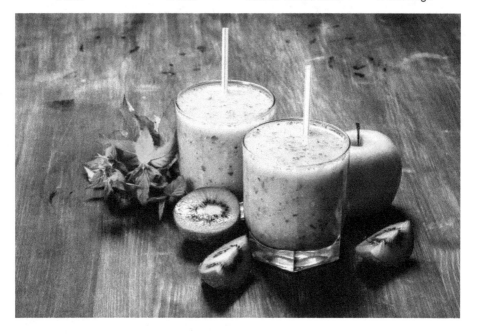

INGREDIENTS

- 1 cup of mango, peeled and cubes
- 1 head of baby romaine lettuce (or spinach), chopped
- 1 kiwi fruit, peeled and diced

DIRECTIONS

1. Blend mango, lettuce and kiwi.

2. Juice apple and cucumber.

3. Next, blend all together.

4. If the taste is strong for you, you may add some water or ice, depending on your preference.

- 1 cucumber, peeled and diced
- 1 medium-sized apple, cored.

NUTRITION (per serving):

Calories: 253 kcal | Fats: 4g | Carbs: 39g | Protein: 18g.

STRAWBERRY-APPLE JUICE DELIGHT

5 min

0 min

Soft & Pureed food

2 Servings

INGREDIENTS

- 1 medium-sized apple, peeled and cored
- 2 cups of strawberries with their tops removed.

DIRECTIONS

1. Juice or blend the strawberries first.
2. Last, blend or juice the apples and mix them with the strawberry juice.

NUTRITION (per serving):

Calories: 120 kcal | Fat: 0g | Carbs: 30g | Protein: 0g.

IMMUNE BOOSTERS

5 min

0 min

Soft & Pureed food

2 Servings

INGREDIENTS

- 1 cup of blueberries
- 2 medium-sized raw beets, cut into quarters
- 1 cup of strawberries, with top ends removed.

DIRECTIONS

1. First, put all the ingredients in a blender.

2. Then blend them until the mixture becomes liquid.

NUTRITION (per serving):

Calories: 10 kcal | Fats: 0g | Carbs: 4g | Protein: 0g.

TROPICAL GREEN PARADISE

5 min

0 min

Soft & Pureed food

2 Servings

INGREDIENTS

- 1 medium-sized cucumber
- 8 to 10 pieces of celery stalks
- 1 small-sized honeydew.

DIRECTIONS

1. Put all the ingredients together in a blender.

2. Then blend them until a liquid consistency is achieved.

NUTRITION (per serving):

Calories: 15 kcal | Fats: 0g |Carbs: 6g | Protein: 0g.

AFTERNOON SUNSHINE

5 min

0 min

Soft & Pureed food

2 Servings

A serving of afternoon sunshine is sure to boost your energy during your admission.

INGREDIENTS

- 1 ripe banana, chopped
- 6 cubes fat-free soy milk
- 6 cubes of fat-free skim milk.

DIRECTIONS

1. Put all the ingredients together in a blender.

2. Then blend them until a liquid consistency is achieved.

NUTRITION (per serving):

Calories: 80 kcal | Fats: 1g | Carbs: 17g | Protein: 0g.

PINK REFRESHER

10 min

0 min

Soft & Pureed food

2 Servings

INGREDIENTS

- 2 cups of watermelon
- 1 cup of cucumber
- 1 cup of water.

DIRECTIONS

1. Add water, cucumber, and watermelon in a blender.
2. Mix them until a smooth and liquid consistency is achieved.

NUTRITION (per serving):

Calories: 140 kcal | Fats: 2.5g | Carbs: 27g | Protein: 1g.

PEANUT & BANANA PROTEIN SHAKE

5 min

0 min

Soft & Pureed food

1 Servings

INGREDIENTS

- 1 scoop chocolate flavored whey protein
- ½ banana, peeled and cut
- 1-2 tbsp. peanut butter
- ½ cup ice cubes
- ½ cup water or non-fat milk.

DIRECTIONS

1. Put all the ingredients together in a blender.
2. Then blend them until smooth.

NUTRITION (per serving):

Calories: 113 kcal | Fats: 7g | Carbs: 21g | Protein: 19g.

CREAMY CORN DELIGHT

| 10 min | 5 min | Soft & Pureed food | 4 Servings |

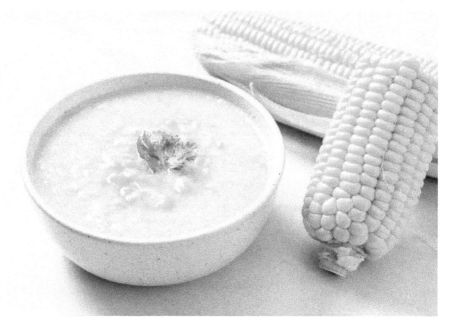

INGREDIENTS

- 3 cups whole kernel corn, canned or boiled
- ½ tbsp. cornstarch
- 3 tbsp. cream of corn powder
- ½ cup evaporated milk

DIRECTIONS

1. Dissolve cream of corn and cornstarch in a half cup of water. Set them aside for a moment.

2. Place the remaining 3½ of water in a cooking pot and heat over medium-high temperature.

3. Next, add all the remaining ingredients to the cooking pot.

- 1 tbsp. vegetable oil
- 2 eggs, beaten
- Salt, to taste
- Ground pepper, to taste
- 4 cups water.

4. Stir until all the ingredients dissolve.

5. Pour in the mixture of cream corn and cornstarch.

6. Heat the cooking pot until it boils.

7. Reduce the temperature and allow it to simmer for 1 to 2 minutes while continually stirring.

8. If you desire a much thinner soup, then add water. Adjust to personal preference, accordingly.

NUTRITION (per serving):

Calories: 107 kcal | Fats: 10g | Carbs: 2g | Protein: 8g.

CAULIFLOWER CHOWDER

15 min

1 h

Soft & Pureed food

6 Servings

INGREDIENTS

- 1 tbsp. olive oil
- 3 cloves garlic, chopped
- 1 medium onion, chopped
- 3 medium carrots, chopped
- 3 cups cauliflower, chopped
- 3½ cups reduced sodium chicken broth
- 1 cup fat-free milk
- ¼ tsp. ground nutmeg
- ½ tsp. basil, dried
- 1 bay leaf
- Salt and pepper, to taste.

DIRECTIONS

1. In a large saucepan, sauté garlic and onion with olive oil until soft over low heat.

2. Add the remaining ingredients except the salt and pepper.

3. Bring to boil and let it simmer over low heat for additional 15 minutes. Season the soup with salt and pepper.

4. Remove from heat.

5. Blend the soup/chowder until smooth.

6. Bring it back to boil until the chowder is thickened. Stir occasionally.

7. Remove from heat. Serve hot.

NUTRITION (per serving):

Calories: 195 kcal | Fats: 7g | Carbs: 31g | Protein: 9.2g.

PUMPKIN SOUP

| 15 min | 40 min | Soft & Pureed food | 6 Servings |

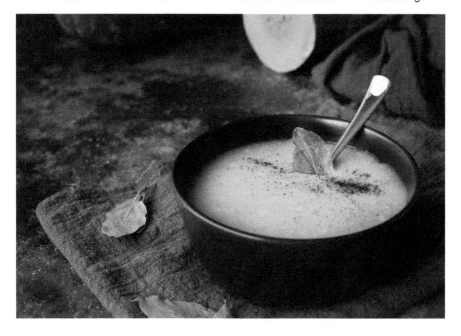

INGREDIENTS

- 1 tbsp. olive oil
- 1 medium onion, chopped
- 4 cloves garlic, minced
- 1 tbsp. ground cumin
- 1 tsp. chili powder

DIRECTIONS

1. In a large pot, sauté onion, garlic, cumin, chili and pepper with olive oil until soft.

2. Add pumpkin puree and broth into the pot. Bring to boil. Stir occasionally.

3. Lower the heat with lid semi uncovered. Let the pumpkin soup

- ½ tsp. ground black pepper
- 2 cups vegetable broth
- 1 can (16 oz) of pumpkin purée (or roasted pumpkin).

simmer over low heat for 25 minutes.

4. Remove from heat. Use a blender to smoothen consistency.

5. Serve hot and enjoy!

NUTRITION (per serving):

Calories: 230 kcal | Fats: 7g | Carbs: 35g | Protein: 9.8g.

KALE & RED LENTIL SOUP

| 10 min | 45 min | Soft & Pureed food | 6 Servings |

This Lentil Kale Soup is nutritious, delicious, vegan and protein-packed.

It's made with simple vegetables like onions, celery and carrots, loaded with plant-protein rich lentils and then finished off with some kale.

INGREDIENTS

- 1 tbsp. extra-virgin olive oil
- 1 cup onion, chopped
- ½ cup carrots, cut into ½-inch chunks
- ½ cup celery, cut into ¼-inch chunks
- 1 tsp. minced garlic
- 1 cup red lentils
- 1 tsp. thyme, dried
- 1 tsp. cumin, ground

DIRECTIONS

1. In a large stock pot over medium heat, heat the olive oil. Add the onion, carrots, celery, and garlic, and sauté until tender, 5 to 7 minutes.

2. Add the lentils, thyme, and cumin. Mix well and stir for 1 to 2 minutes until all the ingredients are coated well with the seasonings.

3. Add the broth and water to the pot. Bring to a simmer, add the kale, and stir well.

4. Add the bay leaf, then cover the pot and simmer for 30 to 35

- 2 cups low-sodium vegetable broth
- 2 cups water
- 2 large stalks kale, stemmed, with leaves chopped (about 2 cups)
- 1 bay leaf
- 2 tbsp. freshly squeezed lemon juice
- Low-fat plain Greek yogurt (optional).

minutes.

5. Remove the pot from the heat.

6. Remove and discard the bay leaf.

7. Stir in the lemon juice.

8. Use an immersion blender to puree the soup to your desired consistency. Alternatively, let the soup cool for 10 minutes before pureeing it in batches in a blender.

9. Garnish each bowl of soup with a dollop of the Greek yogurt (if using) and serve.

NUTRITION (per serving):

Calories: 170 kcal | Fats: 3g | Carbs: 24g | Protein: 13g.

CHEESY BROCCOLI SOUP

10 min

20 min

Soft & Pureed food

8 Servings

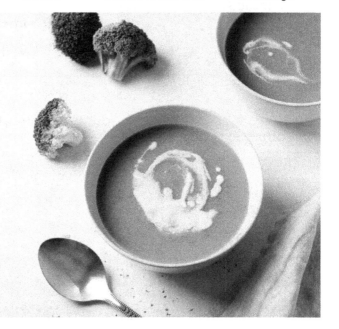

INGREDIENTS

- 1 tbsp. virgin olive oil
- 1 medium onion, chopped
- 1 tbsp. garlic, minced
- 2 cups carrots, grated

DIRECTIONS

1. In a stock pot, heat the olive oil over medium heat. Add the onion and garlic. Stir until fragrant, about 1 minute.

2. Add the carrots and continue to stir until tender, about 2 to 3 minutes. Add the nutmeg and the flour. Continue to cook, stirring

- ¼ tsp. ground nutmeg
- ¼ cup whole-wheat pastry flour
- 2 cups low-sodium vegetable broth
- 2 cups nonfat or 1% milk
- ½ cup fat-free half-and-half
- 3 cups broccoli florets
- 2 cups Cheddar cheese, shredded extra-sharp.

constantly, until browned, 2 to 3 minutes.

3. Add the broth and then the milk and whisk constantly until it starts to thicken. Add the half-and-half and mix to combine well.

4. Stir in the broccoli florets. Bring to a boil and then reduce the heat to a simmer. Cook for 10 minutes or until the broccoli is tender.

5. Use an immersion blender to puree it to a smooth consistency, if desired, or leave it as is for a chunky soup.

6. Stir in the Cheddar cheese until melted. Reserve some cheese as a topping for serving time. Refrigerate any leftovers and eat within 1 week.

NUTRITION (per serving):

Calories: 193 kcal | Fats: 9g | Carbs: 17g | Protein: 12g.

CREAMY TOMATO SOUP DELUXE WITH NAVY BEANS

6 h 15 min

2 h

Soft & Pureed food

4 Servings

INGREDIENTS

- 1 small can tomato paste
- 1 can tomatoes
- 1 cup navy beans
- 4 cups vegetable broth
- 2 tbsp. olive oil
- 3 medium-sized carrots, peeled and then finely chopped
- 1 large-sized leek, chopped thinly
- 1 tbsp. salt
- 2 to 4 cloves garlic, thinly sliced
- 3 tbsp. raw honey

DIRECTIONS

1. First is to soften the beans by soaking them in cold water for 6 hours.

2. After the beans have softened, drain and rinse the beans. Replace it with another set of cold water that's 3 times more than the first batch of water.

3. Place the beans in a large cooking pot and boil over medium-high heat.

4. Once it reached boiling point, turn the heat down by a notch and allow it to simmer. Cooking the beans may take up to 90 minutes.

5. After the beans are tenderized, drain the water and rinse the beans with cold water. Set them

- 2 cups kale, finely chopped
- 1 tbsp. dried dill.

aside for a moment.

6. Place olive oil in cooking oil and heat over medium-high heat. Add in carrots and leeks and pour in 1 tablespoon of salt. And then cook it for roughly 5 to 8 minutes, or until the leeks dehydrate.

7. Add the garlic and cook for another 2 to 3 minutes until it provides a strong fragrance.

8. Next is to add vegetable broth, tomato paste, tomatoes, and dill. Stir them together until the mixture is thoroughly diluted.

9. Again, turn the heat up a notch to induce a gentle boil.

10. Once it boiled, turn it down again to a simmer. Cook for about 15 minutes until the vegetables are tender.

11. Now, add kale, honey, and the beans we cooked earlier. Stir the mixture thoroughly.

12. Cook for 3 to 4 minutes until kale is soft.

13. Transfer 2/3 of the mixture in a separate bowl and use an

immersion blender. Blend until a smooth and liquid consistency is attained.

14. Add the unblended 1/3 part of the mixture into the blended one. When mixed properly, it will present a creamy and silky texture.

15. Put the cooking pot back in the heat. Heat them for a few minutes to allow the flavors to sync.

16. Garnish it with tiny amounts of peanut butter or olive oil. And then with parmesan cheese or herb spices or feta.

NUTRITION (per serving):

Calories: 157.3 kcal | Fats: 1.7g | Carbs: 8g | Protein: 6.7g.

SIMPLE CREAMY GUACAMOLE

15 min

0 min

Soft & Pureed food

2 Servings

INGREDIENTS

- 1 ripe avocado, seeded and peeled
- 1 garlic clove, minced
- 1 tsp. lime or lemon juice
- ¼ tomato, finely chopped
- 1 tbsp. onion, chopped
- 1 tbsp. fresh cilantro leaves
- Salt, to taste.

DIRECTIONS

1. Put all the ingredients together in a blender.

2. Then blend them until smooth.

3. Serve immediately or refrigerate for an hour for best flavor.

NUTRITION (per serving):

Calories: 109 kcal | Fats: 10g | Carbs: 6g | Protein: 1g.

TURKEY CHILI

5 min

25 min

Soft & Pureed food

6 Servings

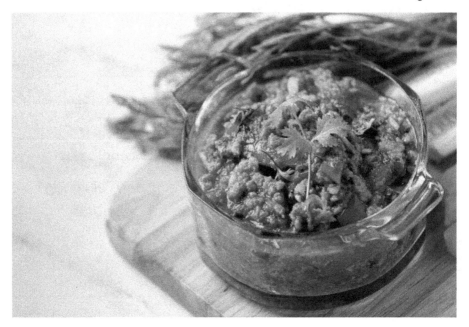

INGREDIENTS

- 1 lb. lean turkey meat, grounded
- 1½ tbsp. chilli powder
- 1 cup chicken broth
- 2 tbsp. olive oil
- 1 medium-sized

DIRECTIONS

1. Place olive oil in a cooking pot and heat over medium temperature.

2. Sauté the onions and cook until softened.

3. Then add the turkey along with the spices.

4. Sauté until the turkey becomes

- onion, finely chopped
- 1½ tsp. cumin
- 1 can (or 28 oz.) pressed tomatoes
- 1 can kidney beans, rinsed and drained
- Ground pepper, to taste
- Salt, to taste.

brown.

5. Next, add the chicken broth and pressed tomatoes.

6. Close the lid of the cooking pot and cook for about 10 minutes.

7. Once the mixture obtains a pureed consistency, add the kidney beans and stir until it is softened.

8. Season it with ground pepper and a tiny pinch of salt.

NUTRITION (per serving):

Calories: 335 kcal | Fats: 6.6g | Carbs: 41.3g | Protein: 21g.

CHEDDAR CHEESE PUFF

| 5 min | 1 h | Soft & Pureed food | 6 Servings |

A flavorful, easy and soft cheesy protein meal that works for breakfast, lunch, supper, or as a tapas style appetizer! Melty cheddar provides the winning flavor for a make ahead bariatric-friendly meal your entire family will love.

INGREDIENTS

- 8 large eggs
- ⅓ cup flour
- 1 tsp. baking powder
- ½ tsp. salt
- Black pepper, to taste
- 1 cup, small curd low fat cottage cheese
- 1 cup Cheddar cheese, shredded
- 2 tbsp. butter, melted.

DIRECTIONS

1. Preheat the oven to 325°F.

2. Beat eggs until light and lemon colored - using an electric hand mixer if desired.

3. Add flour, baking powder, salt, a few grinds of black pepper and blend until smooth.

4. Fold in the cottage cheese, Cheddar cheese and butter.

5. Spray 8x8-inch glass baking dish with nonstick vegetable spray. Pour mixture into the baking dish.

6. Bake for 45 to 50 minutes, until edges are slightly puffed, and the very center of the puff still jiggles a

bit when you move the baking dish.

7. DO NOT OVERBAKE - for a moist cheesy texture, remove from oven when slightly underbaked as the heat will continue to cook it out of the oven.

8. Allow to cool for 10 minutes.

9. Cut into squares and serve.

NUTRITION (per serving):

Calories: 243 kcal | Fats: 19g | Carbs: 9.5g | Protein: 21g.

EGG CUSTARD WITH BERRIES

| 5 min | 50 min | Soft & Pureed food | 4 Servings |

Egg Custard is a wonderful delicious soft dish of cool vanilla creaminess and berry flavor. Easy smooth and creamy. It is the most perfect bariatric food for all post ops.

INGREDIENTS

- 2 large-sized eggs
- 1 cup blueberries
- 1 cup raspberries
- ¼ tsp. nutmeg
- 1 tsp. vanilla extract
- 4 tsp. sugar substitute
- 1 cup water
- 2 cups evaporated milk, nonfat
- ¼ tsp. salt.

DIRECTIONS

1. Heat the oven until it reached 350°F.

2. Pour in water in a baking pan with a measurement of 9x13 inches.

3. Also, prepare an 8x8 baking dish and spray it with nonstick cooking spray.

4. Prepare a small bowl, then place sugar substitute, a pinch of salt, vanilla extract, and eggs.

5. Beat them thoroughly until all ingredients are diluted.

6. Next is to pour the nonfat evaporated milk. Stir the mixture until blended well.

7. Mix and shake raspberries and

blueberries. And then place them at the bottom of the 8x8 baking pan—spread them evenly throughout.

8. Then put the egg mixture on top.

9. Next, transfer the ingredients of the 8x8 pan into the water-filled 9x13 pan.

10. Bake and wait for another 35 minutes, or until no crumbs are sticking to the knife when you put it in.

11. Remove the baking pan from the oven.

12. Lastly, sprinkle nutmeg on top of the custard.

NUTRITION (per serving):

Calories: 140 kcal | Fats: 5g | Carbs: 45g | Protein: 14.2g.

COTTAGE CHEESE FLUFF

10 min	0 min	Soft & Pureed food	4 Servings

INGREDIENTS

- 24 oz. fat-free cottage cheese
- 4 oz. sugar-free whipped crème
- 1 (0.3 oz.) packages sugar-free gelatin, flavor of choice
- Fruits (optional).

DIRECTIONS

1. Mix all ingredients in a medium bowl.

2. Optional — add your favorite fruit pureed in a blender.

NUTRITION (per serving):

Calories: 220 kcal | Fats: 3g | Carbs: 24g | Protein: 22g.

PUMPKIN YOGURT WITH EXTRA KICK

10 min

0 min

Soft & Pureed food

2 Servings

INGREDIENTS

- ½ cup pumpkin, canned
- ¼ tsp. cinnamon
- ⅛ tsp. all-spice
- ⅛ tsp. nutmeg
- ⅛ tsp. ground ginger
- 1 cup vanilla yogurt (light)
- 1 tsp. vanilla extract
- Stevia, to taste
- ½ tsp. liquid butter extract.

DIRECTIONS

1. Combine all ingredients and mix thoroughly.
2. Place in a refrigerator and chill for a few minutes before serving.

NUTRITION (per serving):

Calories: 30 kcal | Fats: 0.1g | Carbs: 8g | Protein: 2g.

PROTEIN POPSICLES

5 min

0 min

Soft & Pureed food

4 Servings

INGREDIENTS

- 2 cups fresh or frozen strawberries, washed and stem removed
- 1 medium ripe banana, peeled and sliced
- 1 cup of pre-made clear protein drinks of your choice.

DIRECTIONS

1. Blend all the ingredients together until smooth.

2. Divide the mixture equally in popsicles mold.

3. Freeze overnight.

NUTRITION (per serving):

Calories: 57 kcal | Fats: 2g | Carbs: 25g | Protein: 26g.

INTRODUCING REAL FOODS

HOW MUCH CAN I EAT AFTER SURGERY?

Now that we have had a chance to talk about some of the basics of this diet plan and how it works, it is time for us to dive into the amount of food or how much we can put into a serving when the surgery is done.

We want to be able to lose weight, so obviously the serving sizes need to be smaller, but we want to make sure that we are eating enough to meet our nutrition needs while not eating so much that we are going to end up straining the stomach and causing injury after this kind of surgery.

When the surgery is done, you want to make sure that you are careful with the amount that you are eating. During the liquid phase and the time before the diet where you are not supposed to eat at all, hopefully, you will start to recognize the difference between having cravings and wanting to eat versus being hungry and actually needing to eat. The more that you are able to learn how to do that, the easier the weight loss will be, and the easier it is for the recovery time after the sleeve as well.

With this in mind, we need to take it slowly and learn how to listen to our bodies. Going back to some of the old ways of doing things and our old eating habits will be hard to do here because the sleeve is going to slow that down. But if you are not careful, over time, the stomach will stretch out, and you will start to take on more food than you should, and the weight will come back. That is why we need to learn how to listen to our bodies and what they tell us as early as possible.

During the first few weeks, you do not have to worry as much about the portions as you will with the other parts. This is the time where you are mostly going to have water and not much else. Your goal is to give the stomach some time to heal, and lots of water is going to be your best friend. Towards the second week, you are able to add in some light things, think the foods you would eat when suffering from a big cold, and the amounts that you would eat during that time as well. But during that first week, you will focus on keeping just with the liquids and maybe some broth if you are feeling a bit hungry.

During the second week, you will not increase your food amounts that much either. You will be allowed to add in a few things like yogurt, pudding, and maybe even a few easy to consume soups as long as they have a ton of nutrition in them. The servings need to stay pretty small. Think like one small pudding cup for breakfast, one small yogurt for lunch, and a kid's bowl of soup for supper, followed with water for the rest of the day. And that is only if you feel up to it. If even that much food is still not sitting well with you, then taper it back and keep things small.

After those first few weeks, your stomach should be feeling better, and if you followed the diet in the right manner you will then be able to increase your portions a bit and eat a little bit more. But you still need to be careful and worry about what is going to feel the best for you here.

The foods that you eat during this time need to be soft and easy to digest because you are only a bit past that mark of having the surgery, and you want to make sure that your stomach is getting the healing that it needs. Lots of soft fruits and vegetables are encouraged here, and just having a little bit is a good place to start. If you are worried about servings, a good idea is to replace all of your dishes, at least for now, with some of the plates that are made for toddlers. The ones that separate out into a few sections can be even better.

This way you can fill up that little plate and know when you are done and should not eat anymore. These will keep some of the meals that you consume down to a minimum and will make it easier for some self-control. In these weeks, your body will be adjusting to some of the changes that you have made, and you want to make sure that you aren't overloading it too much. Starting with some smaller portions is a great way to make sure that we are going to keep our bodies healthy, get the nutrients that we need, and allow for the rest of the healing that is needed.

As you are eating during this stage, and any of the other stages that you work with, you want to make sure that you are eating nice and slow. If you scarf down the meal, you risk eating too much along the way, and you are going to definitely feel it when the time is all done. This is not a healthy way to eat whether you are on this kind of diet plan or not, so avoid it as much as possible and build up some slower eating habits.

It is recommended, especially in the beginning, that you chew your food 25 times before swallowing. If you are still in the first few weeks of eating solid foods, although this may be a bit hard to do with some blended and pureed foods, so don't worry about that as much. But taking your time is going to be so important when you work on this kind of plan and being careful with not scarfing down the food will allow you time to know when you are hungry and can reduce complications from eating too much and tearing the stomach.

If it is too hard to eat the food and take in that many bites at a time, then set a timer for how long you will take to eat the meal. Maybe give yourself 20 minutes to get the plate done. If you feel full before that time, then stop eating, no matter how much is already on the plate still, but make sure that the plate is not empty before the timer goes off.

During this time, you should only eat three meals a day, and the snacking should definitely be limited as much as possible. This will ensure that you are not going to end up with issues of grazing and eating too much as the day goes on and that you can monitor your calories as you go. As you get more familiar with this eating plan, and you are sure that you can handle it all, you can then go through and add in some more foods and meals as well, and maybe have a snack on occasion.

But in the beginning, stick with the three meals a day and do not go back for seconds, or you could cause issues.

Eating is going to be a bit trickier to manage when you are on this kind of diet plan compared to some of the others that you may have done in the past. You are not only learning how to cut down the calories and listen to your body for the actual hunger cues that will tell you when to eat.

You also need to worry about the healing process and not eat too much as you go through this. All of that combined is going to be a bit harder to stick with when you first get started, but it can be a great way to ensure that you can lose weight and keep that weight off for the long term as well.

SOLID FOODS

(From 2 to 3 months and onwards) After 2 or 3 months, you can go back to eating solid foods. But after such, you can feel changes in your appetite and find that you become full quicker before the surgery. Although you may eat more solid foods at this point, it doesn't mean that you're allowed to somewhat careless in what you eat. The following are some examples of foods that are still off-limits during this phase:

- Tough meat – be sure to tenderize or marinade them before consuming.
- Bread – we prefer for you to toast and slice them first.
- High-fat and high-calorie milk products – we advise low-lactose milk and soya milk instead.

Important notes:

- Strictly comply with the diet guidelines provided by your dietician or surgeon.
- Stop eating as soon as you feel full.
- Take time to consume your meals.
- Chew your foods thoroughly.
- Opt for chewable dietary supplements. However, in events, you can't find any crush tablet supplements or pour in water if in capsule form.
- Never skip meals. Eat three times a day.

You may still experience nausea and vomiting from time to time. But as soon as you start experiencing them, stop eating.

BREAKFAST RECIPES

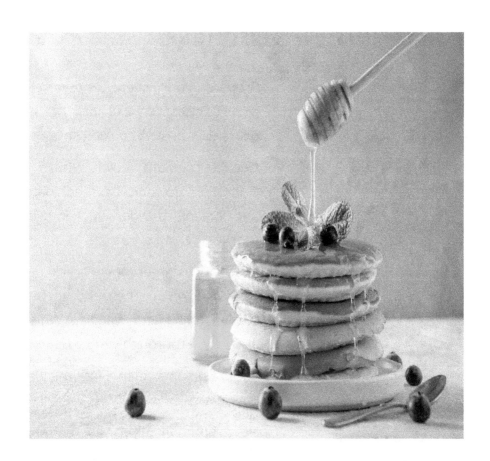

CHERRY-VANILLA BAKED OATMEAL

10 min

45 min

Breakfast

6 Servings

INGREDIENTS

- 3 medium eggs
- 1 cup old-fashioned oats
- 1 tbsp. flaxseed powder
- 1 tsp. vanilla extract
- ½ tsp. cinnamon powder
- 1 cup low-fat milk
- 1 tsp. liquid stevia
- ¾ tsp. baking powder
- 1 medium apple, diced cored and skinless
- ½ cup low-fat plain Greek yogurt

DIRECTIONS

1. Prepare your oven. Preheat to 375°F. Grease an 8x8 inch baking dish with nonstick cooking spray.

2. Get a medium bowl. Pour in cinnamon powder, flaxseed, oats, and baking powder into it. Mix thoroughly and set aside.

3. In a much larger bowl, crack the eggs and whisk. Then add yogurt, stevia, milk, and vanilla. Whisk again until thoroughly mixed.

4. Stir the dry ingredients into the wet ingredients.

5. Now pour in diced apples and cherries, then gently fold them into the mixture.

6. Pour mixture into the prepared baking dish and slide it into the

- 1 cup fresh cherries with the pits removed
- Nonstick cooking spray.

oven to bake.

7. Leave it for about 45 minutes or until you notice the edges pulling away from the walls of the pan and the oatmeal bouncing back when poked.

8. Place any leftovers into airtight glass bowls and place them in the fridge. They will keep for a week. Microwave before serving

Notes: Play around with the extras in the oatmeal. In fact, make the recipes seasonal even. Change it up every now and then. Use pumpkin puree in place of the yogurt. Use unsweetened dried cranberries instead of the usual cherries if you'd like a nice holiday twist. Place the apples and cherries on the shelf and replace them with 100% natural fresh berries. If you would like a super creamy consistency, you can add a quarter cup of low-fat milk when serving.

NUTRITION (per serving):

Calories: 149 kcal | Fats: 4g | Carbs: 21g | Protein: 8g.

HIGH-PROTEIN PANCAKES

5 min

5 min

Breakfast

4 Servings

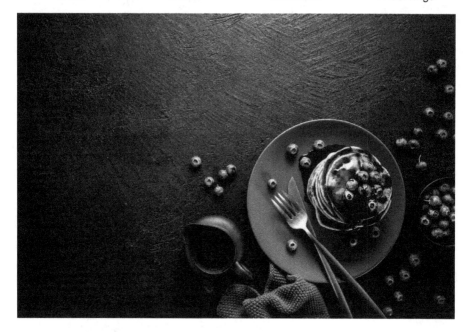

INGREDIENTS

- 1½ tbsp. melted coconut oil
- 3 medium eggs
- ⅓ cup whole wheat pastry flour
- 1 cup low-fat cottage cheese
- Nonstick cooking

DIRECTIONS

1. Gently beat the eggs in a large bowl.

2. Stir in flour, coconut oil, and cottage cheese until thoroughly mixed.

3. Place a large pan over medium-low heat and grease the pan with a single coat of cooking spray.

spray.

4. You will need a measuring cup for this part. Drizzle about ⅓ cup of pancake batter into a greased pan and leave it to cook for about 3 minutes or until you notice air bubbles on top of the pancake.

5. Flip the pancakes to cook the other side until it looks golden brown. This should take about 2 minutes. Take it out of the pan and repeat the process until the batter is finished.

6. Serve warm.

NUTRITION (per serving):

Calories: 182 kcal | Fats: 10g | Carbs: 10g | Protein: 12g.

NO SUGAR YOGURT CAKE

 5 min

 1 h 5 min

 Breakfast

 10 Servings

INGREDIENTS

- ¾ cup almond flour
- ¾ cup all purpose flour
- 2 tsp. baking powder
- ½ tsp. sea salt
- ½ cup Stevia sugar
- ½ cup plain yogurt
- 4 tbsp. butter, melted
- 2 large eggs
- 1 lemon zest, freshly grated
- ½ lemon juice
- 1 tsp. vanilla extract.

DIRECTIONS

1. Preheat oven to 350°F.
1. Coat a loaf pan with non-stick vegetable spray.
2. Whisk together to combine in small bowl the almond flour, flour, baking powder, salt - set aside.
3. In a large bowl, with your fingers, rub together the lemon zest and Stevia.
4. Whisk in the yogurt, butter, eggs, lemon juice and vanilla extract.
5. Blend in the flour mixture.
6. Transfer into loaf pan and smooth top.
7. Bake 40 to 45 minutes, until golden brown, top has risen, and thin skewer inserted near center comes out clean.
8. Let cool on wire rack for 15 minutes, invert onto rack and cool completely.

NUTRITION (per serving):

Calories: 204 kcal | Fats: 23g | Carbs: 17g | Protein: 8.2g.

SOUTHWESTERN SCRAMBLED EGGS BURRITOS

10 min

10 min

Breakfast

8 Servings

INGREDIENTS

- 1 tsp. extra-virgin olive oil
- 1 medium red bell pepper, chopped
- 1 medium green bell pepper, chopped
- ¼ cup low-fat milk
- 8 medium whole wheat tortillas
- 12 small eggs
- 1 can black beans, drained and rinsed
- 1 cup salsa
- ½ medium onion, diced.

DIRECTIONS

1. Mix the eggs and milk in a large bowl.

2. Place a large pan over medium heat and drizzle olive oil onto it.

3. Pour in bell peppers, and onions, then stir-fry for about 3 minutes or until it softens.

4. Stir in the beans.

5. Pour in the milk mixture and lower the heat to a simmer and gently stir with a silicone spatula for roughly 4 minutes or until the eggs look cooked through and fluffy.

6. Place the tortillas on a clean flat surface and scoop the scrambled egg mixture onto each of them.

7. Fold the tortilla. Bottom end first,

then the sides, then roll.

8. Serve warm with a side of salsa.

Notes: Place any leftovers in the fridge to preserve. This will keep for a week. To serve, microwave for 1 minute and 30 seconds.

If you want to store them for longer than a week, you will have to put them on ice.

NUTRITION (per serving):

Calories: 250 kcal | Fats: 10g | Carbs: 28g | Protein: 19g.

HANGRY EGGS

10 min

20 min

Breakfast

6 Servings

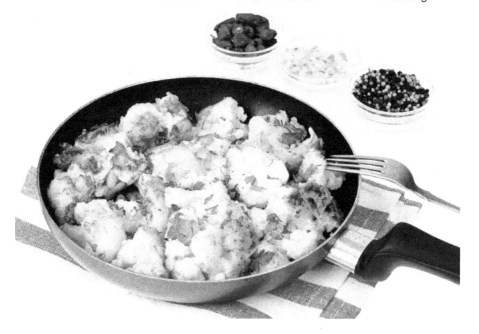

INGREDIENTS

- 2 eggs
- 4 slices deli ham
- ½ bag cauliflower florets
- Cooking spray.

DIRECTIONS

1. Place the cauliflower and 2 tablespoons of water into a bowl and cover in the microwave for 4 minutes to make tender.

1. In the last half a minute, add the ham to this and heat it through. If there is water left, drain it out when you are done.

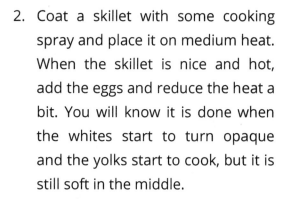

2. Coat a skillet with some cooking spray and place it on medium heat. When the skillet is nice and hot, add the eggs and reduce the heat a bit. You will know it is done when the whites start to turn opaque and the yolks start to cook, but it is still soft in the middle.

3. Place the cauliflower on a plate and have the ham on top. Add the eggs over it all, and then serve.

NUTRITION (per serving):

Calories: 109 kcal | Fats: 4g | Carbs: 6g | Protein: 11g.

GRUYÈRE & PARMESAN SOUFFLÉ

25 min

35 min

Breakfast

5 Servings

INGREDIENTS

- 4 large eggs, separate the yolks from the whites
- 2½ tbsp. unsalted butter
- 3 tbsp. flour
- ½ tsp. garlic powder
- ½ tsp. salt
- ½ tsp. cream of tartar
- ⅛ tsp. black pepper
- ¼ tsp. dry mustard powder
- Pinch of nutmeg
- 1 cup nonfat milk

DIRECTIONS

1. Preheat the oven to 375°F. Grease the ramekin with butter. Set aside.

2. Warm milk in a saucepan over medium-low heat right before boiling. Do not burn the milk.

3. Make the roux (butter and flour mixture): Melt butter in a saucepan over medium heat. Add flour and whisk until mixture begins to bubble, do not allow mixture to brown. Remove saucepan from heat.

4. Let the roux stand for few minutes to cool. Pour in warm milk, whisking until smooth. Return to heat.

5. Whisk the mixture of roux and milk constantly until thick, for about 2 to

- 1 cup low-fat Gruyère (or Cheddar, or Swiss cheese), shredded
- ½ cup Parmesan, shredded.

3 minutes. Remove from heat.

6. Add black pepper, salt, and nutmeg. Add egg yolks one at a time, whisking to blend after each addition.

7. Scrape the mixture into large bowl and let it rest at room temperature.

8. Use a mixer to beat egg whites in another large bowl for 3 minutes. Then add cream of tartar, mix again until the egg whites form a stiff peak.

9. Fold ¼ of whites into lukewarm or room temperature mixture. Do not over mix. Add the cheese along with egg whites.

10. Transfer the soufflé mixture to prepared ramekin.

11. Place ramekin in the oven for 35 minutes or until soufflé is puffed and golden brown on top. Do not open the oven for the first 20 minutes or the batter will deflate.

NUTRITION (per serving):

Calories: 312 kcal | Fats: 27.1g | Carbs: 15.4g | Protein: 22.8g.

OMELET IN A CUP

5 min

5 min

Breakfast

1 Servings

INGREDIENTS

- 1 large egg
- 1 tbsp. water
- Salt and paper, to taste
- Cooking spray.

DIRECTIONS

12. Lightly coat a microwave-safe cup with cooking spray.

13. In a cup, beat egg, water, salt and pepper with a fork. Mix well.

14. Cook in a microwave for 60 seconds or until egg is fully cooked.

NUTRITION (per serving):

Calories: 109 kcal | Fats: 4g | Carbs: 6g | Protein: 11g.

ENTREE & SNACK RECIPES

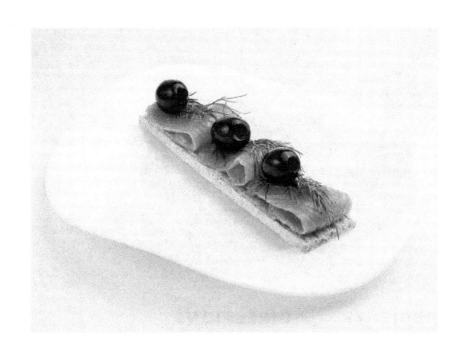

CAPRESE SALAD BITES

10 min   15 min   Entrees & Snacks   12 Servings

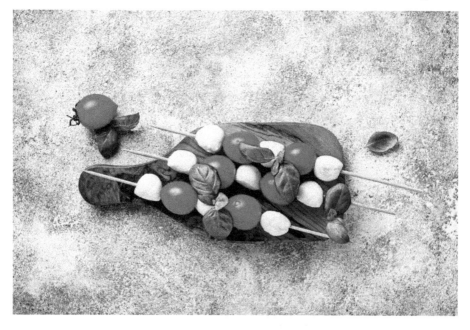

INGREDIENTS

- 24 cherry tomatoes
- 12 mozzarella balls
- 12 fresh basil leaves.

For the Balsamic Glaze

DIRECTIONS

TO MAKE THE BITES

1. Using 12 toothpicks or short skewers, assemble each with 1 cherry tomato, 1 mozzarella ball, 1 basil leaf, and another tomato.

2. Place on a serving platter or in a

- ½ cup balsamic vinegar
- 2 tbsp. extra-virgin olive oil
- 1 garlic clove, minced
- 1 tsp. Italian seasoning.

large glass storage container that can be sealed.

TO MAKE THE GLAZE

3. In a small saucepan, bring the balsamic to a simmer. Simmer for 15 minutes, or until syrupy. Set aside to cool and thicken.

4. In a small bowl, whisk olive oil, garlic, Italian seasoning, and cooled vinegar.

5. Drizzle the olive oil and balsamic glaze over the skewers. Serve immediately or keep in the refrigerator for a tasty snack.

NUTRITION (per serving):

Calories: 23 kcal | Fats: 2g | Carbs: 0.4g | Protein: 2g.

SHRIMP STUFFED AVOCADOS

15 min

2 min

Entrees & Snacks

4 Servings

Shrimp and avocado are a match made in heaven. Beautifully ripe avocado is a fat in this dish - it replaces the mayonnaise!

There is not a recipe for this one as it's that easy!

INGREDIENTS

- 3 average sized avocados, halved
- 1 ib. small shrimp, precooked (40 to 50 count)
- 1 medium Roma tomato, diced very small
- ⅓ medium English cucumber, diced very small
- ⅓ cup red onion, diced very small
- ¼ cup fresh

DIRECTIONS

1. From each avocado half, scoop out about 50% of the flesh and put into a large bowl and mash with a fork. (You want to widen and somewhat hollow out the area to fill the avocado halves so there's space to add the shrimp mixture, but you don't want them totally clean).

2. Add all the other ingredients and stir to combine.

3. Taste the mixture and season with salt, pepper, lime juice, hot sauce, etc. to taste.

4. Spoon the mixture into the

cilantro, finely minced

- 2 to 3 tbsp. lime juice
- Salt, to taste
- Black pepper, to taste
- Hot sauce, to taste.

hollowed out avocados and serve immediately. Recipe is best fresh.

NUTRITION (per serving):

Calories: 313 kcal | Fats: 17g | Carbs: 13g | Protein: 28.5g.

ZUCCHINI MUFFINS

15 min

15 min

Entrees & Snacks

8 Servings

INGREDIENTS

- 4 organic eggs
- ¼ cup unsalted butter, melted
- ¼ cup water
- ⅓ cup coconut flour
- ½ tsp. organic baking powder
- ¼ tsp. salt
- 1½ cups zucchini, grated
- ½ cup Parmesan cheese, shredded
- 1 tbsp. fresh oregano, minced
- 1 tbsp. fresh thyme, minced
- ¼ cup Cheddar

DIRECTIONS

1. Preheat the oven to 400ºF.

2. Lightly, grease 8 muffin tins.

3. Add eggs, butter, and water in a mixing bowl and beat until well combined.

4. Add the flour, baking powder, and salt, and mix well.

5. Add remaining ingredients except for cheddar and mix until just combined.

6. Place the mixture into prepared muffin cups evenly.

7. Bake for approximately 13–15 minutes or until top of muffins become golden-brown.

8. Remove the muffin tin from oven and situate onto a wire rack for 10 minutes.

cheese, grated.

9. Carefully invert the muffins onto a platter and serve warm.

NUTRITION (per serving):

Calories: 187 kcal | Fats: 23g | Carbs: 8.7g | Protein: 13.2g.

CHEESE JALAPENO MUFFINS

10 min

20 min

Entrees & Snacks

12 Servings

INGREDIENTS

- Cooking spray, for pan
- 9 eggs
- 6 bacon slices
- ¾ cup heavy cream
- 1½ jalapeno pepper, sliced
- 8.5 oz. cheddar cheese, shredded
- Pepper
- Salt.

DIRECTIONS

1. Preheat the oven to 350°F. Prep muffin tray with cooking spray and add cooked bacon slices to each muffin cup.

2. In a large bowl, whisk together eggs, cheese, cream, pepper, and salt.

3. Pour egg mixture into the prepared muffin tray.

4. Add sliced jalapeno into each muffin cup.

5. Bake for 15-20 minutes.

NUTRITION (per serving):

Calories: 28 kcal | Fats: 2.4g | Carbs: 1g | Protein: 6.4g.

STUFFED CELERY CRACK

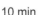

10 min

20 min

Entrees & Snacks

12 Servings

INGREDIENTS

- 1 bunch of celery
- 1 (8-oz.) block cream cheese
- 1 cup dill pickles, chopped
- 1 tbsp. dill pickles juice
- ½ tsp. salt
- 6 crispy bacon strips, chopped
- 3 tbsp. grease
- ¾ tsp. onion powder
- ½ tsp. parsley
- ¾ tsp. garlic powder
- ¼ tsp. dried or fresh dill.

DIRECTIONS

1. Wash the celery and cut it into about 4" pieces (or smaller, as desired).

2. Mix all ingredients below celery together well, then with a spoon begin filling each stalk very well and sprinkle with the dill.

3. Optional: add 1/2 chopped olives, 1/2 chopped pickles and without the bacon.

NUTRITION (per serving):

Calories: 32 kcal | Fats: 3.3g | Carbs: 1g | Protein: 3.4g.

CALIFORNIA ROLL BITES

10 min   0 min   Entrees & Snacks   12 Servings

INGREDIENTS

- 1 English cucumber, cut into 12 ½-inch rounds
- 12 large shrimp, cleaned, cooked and cooled
- 1 large ripe avocado
- Wasabi sauce
- Sriracha sauce.

DIRECTIONS

1. Cut avocado into 12 pieces about the size of your shrimp.

2. Arrange the cucumber slices on a decorative tray, top with a shrimp, avocado piece, a dime sized drop of wasabi sauce, a squeeze of Sriracha sauce.

3. Skewer with a bamboo pick. Enjoy!

NUTRITION (per serving):

Calories: 78 kcal | Fats: 2g | Carbs: 1g | Protein: 11g.

MAIN RECIPES

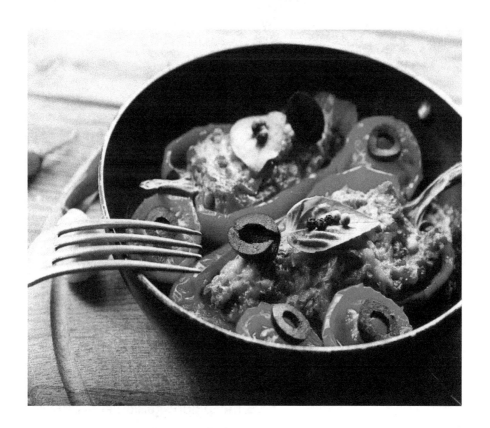

VEGAN SHEPHERD'S PIE

 15 min   45 min   Vegetarian Mains   4 Servings

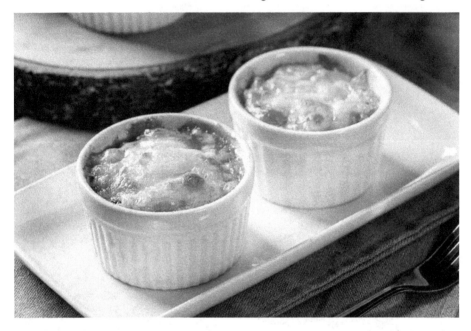

INGREDIENTS

- 1 lb. cooked potatoes, mashed
- 2 tbsp. olive oil
- 1 medium onion, chopped
- 3 garlic cloves, minced
- 1 cup cooked

DIRECTIONS

1. Preheat oven to 425°F.

2. Coat a large skillet with olive oil.

3. Sauté onion, garlic, lentils, thyme, parsley, and frozen vegetables over medium heat for 1-2 minutes.

4. Deglaze the skillet with vegetable stock. Stir well.

lentils

- 1 cup vegetable stock
- 1 tsp. thyme, dried
- 3 tbsp. fresh parsley, chopped
- 2 cups frozen mixed vegetables
- Salt and pepper to taste.

5. Season vegetable mixture with salt and pepper to taste.

6. Divide the vegetable mixture evenly into 4 small ramekins, or heatproof cups.

7. Top the mixture with an even coat of 1-2 tablespoons of mashed potatoes.

8. Bake at 425°F for 15 minutes or until the mashed potatoes on top is lightly golden.

N U T R I T I O N (per serving):

Calories: 194 kcal | Fats: 2.7g | Carbs: 39g | Protein: 9g.

EGGPLANT AND CHICKPEA QUINOA

15 min   20 min   Vegetarian Mains   8 Servings

INGREDIENTS

- 1 medium red bell pepper, diced
- ¼ tsp. cayenne pepper
- 1 tsp. extra-virgin olive oil
- 2 tsp. smoked paprika
- 4 tsp. garlic, minced
- 1 large onion, chopped
- ½ cup water
- 1 tsp. turmeric powder
- 1 cup chicken and vegetable stock
- 1 medium

DIRECTIONS

1. Drizzle olive oil into a large pan and place it over medium heat. Pour in garlic and stir-fry for about 1 minute.

2. Stir in bell pepper and onion, then continue to stir-fry for about 3 minutes or until soft.

1. Sprinkle turmeric, cayenne pepper, cumin, and smoked paprika. Leave to cook for 2 minutes.

2. Stir in eggplant, tomatoes, chickpeas, squash, and water. Place a lid on the pan and lower the heat just a little bit and let it cook for 15 minutes.

3. Meanwhile, as you wait for the chickpeas and veggies to cook, whip about a saucepan and place it

- eggplant, chopped
- 3 medium tomatoes, chopped
- Low-fat plain greek yogurt
- 1 can chickpeas, drained and rinsed
- 1 medium yellow summer squash, chopped
- ½ cup packaged quinoa.

over medium heat. In goes the stock and quinoa. Cover the saucepan and leave it to boil.

4. Once that happens, lower the heat and allow it to simmer until the quinoa absorbs all the stock. This usually takes about 15 minutes.

5. Take the saucepan off the heat and fluff the quinoa.

6. To serve, scoop some quinoa into a plate and serve with curried vegetables and a scoop of yogurt.

NUTRITION (per serving):

Calories: 131 kcal | Fats: 2g | Carbs: 23g | Protein: 6g.

CHICKPEAS CURRY

15 min

20 min

Vegetarian Mains

8 Servings

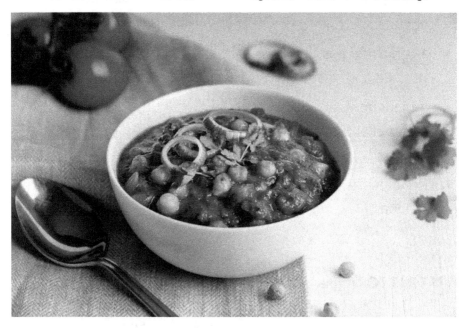

INGREDIENTS

- 1 (15 oz.) cans chickpeas, rinsed and drained
- 1 tbsp. olive oil
- 1 large onion, chopped
- 1 garlic clove, minced

DIRECTIONS

1. In a cooking pan, heat the olive oil over medium heat. Add chopped onion. Stir until the onion is softened and starting to brown.

2. Slightly reduce the heat, add garlic, stir for 30 seconds or until fragrant.

3. Stir in the curry powder, cook for additional 30 seconds.

- 1 tbsp. curry powder
- 1 cup vegetable stock
- ¼ cup cilantro, freshly chopped
- Salt and pepper, to taste.

4. Add drained chickpeas and vegetable stock to the pan. Continue to cook and stir all ingredients together.

5. Bring to a boil, reduce the heat, and let it continue to simmer for about 10-15 minutes.

6. Add salt and paper to taste.

7. Turn off the heat and garnish the chickpeas curry with freshly chopped cilantro.

NUTRITION (per serving):

Calories: 177 kcal | Fats: 3g | Carbs: 32g | Protein: 9g.

ZUCCHINI LASAGNA ROLL-UPS

| 30 min | 30 min | Vegetarian Mains | 6 Servings |

INGREDIENTS

- 3 large zucchini, trimmed and sliced lengthwise into -inch-thick strips
- 1 tsp. salt
- Nonstick cooking spray
- 1 (10-ounce) bag fresh spinach
- 1 cup part-skim ricotta
- ½ cup Parmesan cheese
- 1 large egg
- 2 garlic cloves, minced
- 2 tsp. Italian seasoning

DIRECTIONS

1. Preheat the oven to 400°F.
2. Lay the zucchini slices flat on a paper towel-lined baking sheet, and sprinkle with salt. Let sit for 15 minutes.
3. Meanwhile, spray a small skillet with nonstick cooking spray, and set over medium heat. Add the spinach and cook for 2 minutes, or until wilted. Remove from the heat.
4. In a medium bowl, mix the ricotta, Parmesan, egg, garlic, and Italian seasoning until well combined.
5. Pat the zucchini dry, removing excess salt.
6. Spread 1 cup of marinara in the bottom of a 9-by-9-inch baking dish. Spread each zucchini slice with a spoonful of ricotta mixture, then gently roll up and place in the

- 1½ cups marinara sauce
- 1 cup part-skim Mozzarella, shredded.

prepared baking dish, seam-side down. Repeat with the remaining zucchini and filling. Top with the remaining ½ cup of marinara, and sprinkle with the mozzarella cheese.

7. Bake for 25 to 30 minutes, or until the lasagna rolls are heated through, and the cheese begins to brown.
8. Serve immediately.

NUTRITION (per serving):

Calories: 240 kcal | Fats: 13g | Carbs: 16g | Protein: 18g.

SPAGHETTI SQUASH CHOW

10 min

55 min

Vegetarian Mains

3 Servings

A healthier low-carb version of everyone's favorite takeout dish.
Even your picky eaters will love this!
Only 252 kcal/serving!

INGREDIENTS

- Nonstick cooking spray
- 1 small (3-to 4-pound) spaghetti squash
- ¼ cup low-sodium soy sauce
- 3 garlic cloves, minced
- 1 tbsp. oyster sauce
- 1 inch ginger root, peeled and minced
- 2 tbsp. extra-virgin olive oil

DIRECTIONS

1. Preheat the oven to 350°F. Coat a baking sheet with cooking spray.

2. Halve the spaghetti squash, remove and discard the seeds, and place the halves cut side down on the prepared baking sheet. Bake for 30 to 45 minutes, or until the flesh is tender and can be scraped with a fork.

3. Remove from the oven and let cool. Scrape out the flesh with a fork, creating small noodles. Set aside.

4. In a small bowl, whisk together the soy sauce, garlic, oyster sauce, and ginger.

- 1 small white onion, diced
- 3 celery stalks, thinly sliced
- 2 cups shredded cabbage (or coleslaw mix).

5. In a large skillet over medium heat, heat the oil. Add the onion and celery and cook, stirring, until tender, 3 to 4 minutes.

6. Add the cabbage and cook, stirring, until heated through, 1 to 2 minutes.

7. Add the spaghetti squash and sauce mixture. Continue cooking for another 2 minutes.

8. Serve immediately.

NUTRITION (per serving):

Calories: 252 kcal | Fats: 11g | Carbs: 39g | Protein: 6g.

TOFU STIR-FRY

  15 min

 40 min

 Vegetarian Mains

 4 Servings

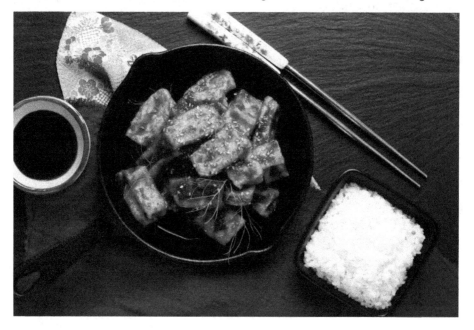

INGREDIENTS

- 1 (14-ounces) block extra-firm tofu
- Nonstick cooking spray
- 1 tbsp. sesame oil
- 3 cups frozen stir-fry vegetable

DIRECTIONS

1. Drain the tofu and wrap in a kitchen towel. Place a plate on top of the tofu, and top with something heavy, such as a book or skillet. Let dry for 15 minutes, changing the towel if necessary.

2. Once dry, chop into 1-inch cubes or rectangles. Arrange the tofu on a

blend

- ½ cup Stir-Fry Sauce.

lightly greased or parchment paper-covered baking sheet, and bake for 25 to 35 minutes, or until golden brown, flipping halfway through. Once golden brown, remove from the oven and let cool while you continue cooking.

3. Heat a large skillet over medium-high heat. Add the sesame oil and swirl to coat. Add the veggies and stir-fry or toss to coat. Cook for 5 minutes.

4. Add the stir-fry sauce and stir to coat. Add the tofu and stir. Cook for 3 to 5 minutes, gently stirring constantly.

5. When the veggies reach the tenderness of your liking, remove from the heat, and serve.

NUTRITION (per serving):

Calories: 163 kcal | Fats: 8g | Carbs: 11g | Protein: 12g.

BLACKENED SALMON WITH AVOCADO CREAM

10 min

10 min

Fish & Seafood
Mains

4 Servings

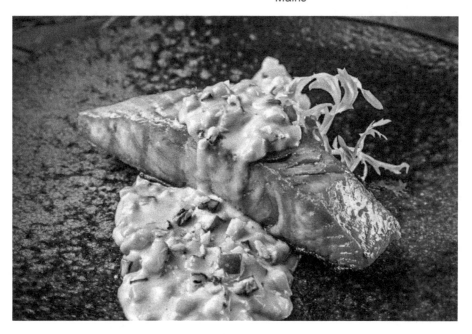

INGREDIENTS

- 4 (6-ounce) salmon fillets, bones removed
- 1 tbsp. butter, melted
- 2 tbsp. blackened

DIRECTIONS

1. Pat the salmon fillets dry on both sides with paper towels.

1. Brush the butter over the fleshy side of the salmon fillets.

2. Pour the seasoning onto a plate and press the flesh side of each

- seasoning
- 1 tbsp. extra-virgin olive oil
- ½ cup Avocado Cream.

salmon fillet into the seasoning, coating evenly.

3. In a large skillet over medium heat, heat the olive oil. Add the salmon, skin-side up, and cook until blackened, 3 to 4 minutes.

4. Flip the fillets and continue to cook to your liking, 5 to 7 minutes, depending on the thickness of the fillets, or to an internal temperature of 125 to 145°F. Once done, the fish should flake easily with a fork.

5. Transfer to individual plates, and serve with the avocado cream.

NUTRITION (per serving):

Calories: 356kcal | Fats: 24g | Carbs: 2g | Protein: 35g.

SHRIMP CEVICHE

10 min

30 min

Fish & Seafood
Mains

4 Servings

INGREDIENTS

- 1 lb. cooked jumbo shrimp
- 1 cup diced tomatoes
- ½ cup finely chopped red onion
- 1 jalapeño pepper, minced
- ¼ cup lemon and lime juice
- ½ cup chopped fresh cilantro
- Salt, to taste
- 1 avocado, pitted and peeled.

DIRECTIONS

1. In a large bowl, mix the shrimp, tomatoes, red onion, and jalapeño.

2. Pour in the lemon and lime juice, cilantro, and salt to taste. Gently toss to coat.

3. For best flavor, cover and refrigerate for at least 30 minutes.

4. Dice the avocado into half-inch chunks right before serving. Add it to the shrimps.

NUTRITION (per serving):

Calories: 207 kcal | Fats: 8g | Carbs: 11g | Protein: 25g.

TUNA PATTIES

5 min

20 min

Fish & Seafood
Mains

8 Servings

INGREDIENTS

- 4 (3-ounces) tuna cans
- 16 cracker pieces, crushed
- 4 egg whites
- ¼ cup carrot, grated
- 1 tbsp. onion, finely sliced
- Dried mustard
- Ground pepper, to taste
- ¼ cup water chestnuts, chopped.

DIRECTIONS

1. Prepare a bowl and mix all the ingredients in one go.
2. Blend them thoroughly using your hands.
3. Form patties. With the ingredients provided above, you can form about 8 patties.
4. Use nonstick cooking spray onto a medium-sized skillet.
5. Heat the skillet over medium temperature.
6. Cook the patties for about 2 to 3 minutes, or until it's golden brown consistency on each side is achieved.

NUTRITION (per serving):

Calories: 130 kcal | Fats: 4,9g | Carbs: 0,3g | Protein: 15,8g.

SHRIMPS WITH TOMATO & FENNEL

 5 min

 25 min

 Fish & Seafood Mains

 4 Servings

INGREDIENTS

- 1 lb. shrimps, peeled & cleaned
- 1 cup fennel, diced
- 1 medium onion, chopped
- 2 garlic cloves, minced
- 1 tbsp. olive oil
- 1 tbsp. tomato paste
- 1 cup white wine (or broth)
- 1 cup tomatoes, crushed
- Red pepper flakes to taste
- Salt and black

DIRECTIONS

1. Sauté fennel, onion, and garlic in olive oil until softened and golden.

2. Stir in tomato paste, add white wine, tomatoes, salt, pepper and a big pinch of crushed red pepper flakes to taste.

3. Bring to a boil, lower heat and allow to reduce for 15 minutes until thickened.

4. Add shrimp and poach until just cooked through. Stir in basil.

5. Serve in a deep bowl with lots of sauce.

pepper

- 4 or 5 basil leaves, minced.

N U T R I T I O N (per serving):

Calories: 196 kcal | Fats: 8g | Carbs: 5g | Protein: 22g.

PAN SEARED COD FILLET

15 min

10 min

Fish & Seafood
Mains

2 Servings

INGREDIENTS

- 2 (3 oz.) Atlantic Cod fillets
- 1 tbsp. olive oil
- 1 garlic clove, minced
- 2 lemon wedges
- 1 branch fresh thyme
- 1 branch fresh rosemary
- Salt and black pepper.

DIRECTIONS

1. Season fillets with minced garlic, a pinch of salt and black pepper. (Optional: sprinkle thyme and rosemary leaves).

2. In a preheated skillet, add 1 tablespoon of olive oil.

3. Place the fish fillets and let it cook for about 2-3 minutes on each side or until fully cooked in the center.

4. Remove fish from heat and serve with lemon wedges if desired.

NUTRITION (per serving):

Calories: 90 kcal | Fats: 1g | Carbs: 2g | Protein: 19g.

MOIST CHICKEN DELUXE

| 15 min | 80 min | Poultry Mains | 12 Servings |

INGREDIENTS

- 3 lb. chicken breasts, boneless and skinless
- 1¼ cups whole wheat Italian breadcrumbs
- ½ cup light mayonnaise dressing.

DIRECTIONS

1. Heat the oven over 425°.

2. Using a culinary brush, apply mayonnaise to the chicken breasts.

3. Put Italian breadcrumbs into a separate plate and roll the chicken breasts over it until fully coated.

4. Next, use an aluminum foil pan and place the chicken breasts. Bake for about 40 to 45 minutes, or until the meat temperature reaches 165°F

NUTRITION (per serving):

Calories: 320 kcal | Fats: 6g | Carbs: 41,3g | Protein: 28g.

TURKEY MEATBALLS SOUP

30 min

35 min

Poultry Mains

8 Servings

INGREDIENTS

FOR TURKEY
MEATBALLS

- 1 lb. lean ground turkey
- 1 egg
- ½ cup grated Parmesan cheese
- 2 tbsp. fresh basil, chopped
- 2 garlic cloves, minced
- ¾ tsp. salt
- ¼ tsp. ground black pepper

FOR BROTH

- 8 cups low-sodium chicken broth
- 1 cup carrots, peeled and sliced

DIRECTIONS

1. Combine egg, turkey, Parmesan cheese, garlic, basil, salt and pepper in medium sized bowl.

2. Shape the turkey mixture by hand into meatballs. Place shaped meatballs on baking sheet or plate. Let them chill for 30 minutes.

3. While waiting for the meatballs to chill, bring chicken broth to boil, add carrots, celery, and onions. Reduce the heat and let it simmer semi- uncovered for 10 minutes.

4. Add the chilled turkey meatballs. Simmer for another 10-15 minutes. Make sure the meatballs are cooked thoroughly.

5. Stir in the parsley leaves.

6. Season with salt and pepper to taste.

- 1 cup celery, sliced
- ¼ bunch parsley leaves, chopped
- ½ medium onion, chopped.

NUTRITION (per serving):

Calories: 169 kcal | Fats: 4.8g | Carbs: 12.6g | Protein: 17.9g.

CHICKEN & BEAN SOUP

5 min

35 min

Poultry Mains

6 Servings

Lots of great flavors pulled from the shelves and quickly combined in this stew.
This makes plenty for a supper plus either lunches or freeze for another meal!

INGREDIENTS

- 1 sweet onion, diced
- 2 garlic cloves, finely chopped
- 1 tbsp. olive oil
- 1¼ lb. chicken thighs, boneless and skinless, each cut into 4 pieces
- 1 tbsp. smoked sweet paprika
- Sea salt and black pepper, to taste
- 1 cup chicken broth

DIRECTIONS

1. Sauté the onion and garlic in the olive oil over medium high heat in a heavy large, covered skillet until softened, 2 to 4 minutes.

1. Season the chicken with half of the paprika, salt and pepper and add to the pan with the onions.

2. Cook until browned, 4 to 6 minutes.

3. Stir in the rest of the paprika and then add the broth, tomatoes, roasted peppers, beans and artichokes.

4. Reduce heat cover and simmer 20 to 25 minutes, until chicken is tender.

- 1 (15-ounce) can diced (fire roasted) tomatoes
- 1 (6-ounce) jar roasted red peppers, sliced
- 1 (15-ounce) can pinto beans, drained and rinsed
- 1 (5-ounce) jar marinated artichoke quarters, drained
- ¼ cup green olives with pimento
- Chopped flat leaf parsley.

5. Stir in the olives and parsley.

NUTRITION (per serving):

Calories: 172 kcal | Fats: 4g | Carbs: 10g | Protein: 24g.

CHICKEN MEATLOAF

15 min

40 min

Poultry Mains

1 Loaf

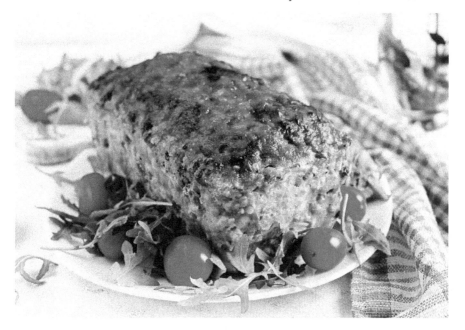

INGREDIENTS

- 1 lb. ground chicken breasts
- ¼ cup onion, minced
- ½ cup breadcrumbs or panko
- 1 egg

DIRECTIONS

1. Preheat the oven to 350°F.

2. Spray the baking dish with oil to prevent sticking.

3. Mix all the ingredients in a large bowl.

4. Add a few tablespoons of chicken broth to make the meatloaf

- ¼ cup celery, minced
- ¼ cup carrot, minced
- 2 cloves garlic, minced
- 3 tbsp. parsley, chopped
- ½ tsp. salt
- ½ tsp. black pepper
- Few tbsp. of chicken broth.

mixture moist but not watery.

5. Transfer the meatloaf mixture to a baking dish. Cook for 40 minutes or until the loaf is fully cooked / inner temperature reach 165°F.

NUTRITION (per serving):

Calories: 124.9 kcal | Fats: 5g | Carbs: 8.6g | Protein: 11.6g.

CHICKEN & ZUCCHINI CASSEROLE

15 min

15 min

Poultry Mains

6 Servings

INGREDIENTS

- 3 medium zucchini, quartered
- 1½ lb. chicken breasts
- 1 (28-oz.) can diced tomatoes
- ½ cup pepperoncini peppers
- ¼ cup black olives, halved
- 1 tsp. Italian seasoning
- Sea salt and black pepper
- 1 cup shredded Italian cheese:

DIRECTIONS

1. Preheat oven to 375°F.

2. Cut zucchini, pepperoncini peppers and chicken breasts into 1-inch cubes. Drain tomatoes.

3. In a large baking dish toss the chicken, zucchini, peppers, olives, Italian seasoning, tomatoes, salt and pepper.

4. Cover with foil and bake for 35 to 45 minutes, until chicken is just cooked through. Remove foil add cheese and bake until cheese is melted, 8 to 10 minutes.

Mozzarella,
Provolone, Fontina
blend.

NUTRITION (per serving):

Calories: 268 kcal | Fats: 20g | Carbs: 11 g | Protein: 12g.

ZOODLES WITH MEAT SAUCE

10 min

40 min

Beef & Pork Mains

4 Servings

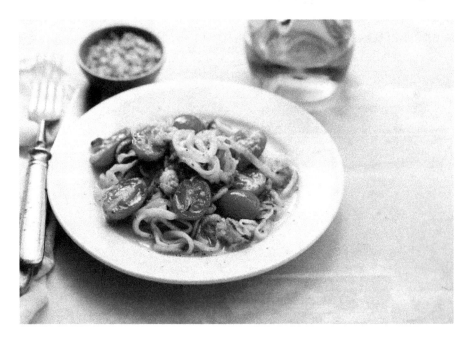

INGREDIENTS

- 1 lb. ground beef (93%)
- 2 tbsp. extra-virgin olive oil
- 1 large yellow onion, chopped
- 3 garlic cloves, minced

DIRECTIONS

1. In a large saucepan over medium heat, cook the ground beef, breaking it up with the spoon, until browned, 7 to 10 minutes. Drain, and transfer to a plate.

2. In the same pan over medium heat, heat 1 tablespoon of oil. Add the onions and garlic, and sauté

- 1 tbsp. tomato paste
- 1 (24-ounce) jar pasta sauce
- 1 tbsp. Italian seasoning
- 4 medium zucchini
- ½ cup Parmesan cheese, shredded.

until the onions are translucent and the garlic is fragrant, about 5 minutes. Add the tomato paste, and sauté for 1 minute.

3. Add the pasta sauce and stir well to combine. Mix in the Italian seasoning. Simmer for 20 minutes.

4. Meanwhile, cut the zucchini noodles to their desired length.

5. In a large skillet over medium heat, heat the remaining tablespoon of oil. Add the zucchini, and sauté until soft, 2 to 3 minutes, or to desired texture. Be sure not to overcook the zucchini, as it will end up mushy.

6. Plate the zucchini, top with the sauce and Parmesan, and serve.

NUTRITION (per serving):

Calories: 410 kcal | Fats: 20g | Carbs: 26g | Protein: 32g.

BEEF STEW WITH RUTABAGA & CARROTS

15 min	40 min	Beef & Pork Mains	3 Servings

This rich, hearty beef stew has a garden full of flavor with vegetables like rutabaga and carrots.
You can throw in extra vegetables to stretch it.

INGREDIENTS

- 4 tsp. extra-virgin olive oil
- 1 lb. beef sirloin steak, cut into 1-inch cubes
- 2 tsp. garlic, minced
- 1 medium onion, chopped
- 1 lb. rutabaga, peeled and cut into ½-inch cubes
- 3 medium carrots, peeled and cut into ½-inch cubes

DIRECTIONS

1. In a large soup pot or Dutch oven, heat 2 teaspoons of olive oil over medium heat.

2. Add the beef and brown it on all sides, stirring frequently, until no longer pink, about 5 minutes. Transfer to a bowl and set aside.

3. In the same pot, heat the remaining 2 teaspoons of olive oil over medium heat. Add the garlic and onion, and cook, stirring frequently, until the onion is tender, 1 to 2 minutes.

4. Stir in the rutabaga, carrots, tomato, paprika, coriander, and

- 1 small tomato, diced
- 1 tsp. smoked paprika
- ½ tsp. ground coriander
- ¼ tsp. red pepper flakes
- 2 tbsp. whole-wheat flour
- ½ cup red wine
- 3 cups low-sodium beef broth
- Fresh minced parsley for garnish.

red pepper flakes.

5. Add the flour and cook, stirring constantly, for 1 minute. Add the red wine and stir for an additional minute.

6. Add the broth and return the beef to the pot. Bring to a boil and then reduce the heat to low to simmer. The sauce should start to thicken.

7. Cover the pot and cook for 30 minutes, or until all the vegetables are tender.

8. Serve garnished with the parsley.

NUTRITION (per serving):

Calories: 292 kcal | Fats: 13g | Carbs: 8g | Protein: 34g.

ONE-PAN PORK CHOPS WITH APPLES & RED ONION

10 min

30 min

Beef & Pork Mains

4 Servings

INGREDIENTS

- 2 tsp. extra-virgin olive oil
- 4 boneless center-cut thin pork chops
- 2 small apples, thinly sliced
- 1 small red onion, thinly sliced
- 1 cup low-sodium chicken broth
- 1 tsp. Dijon mustard
- 1 tsp. dried sage
- 1 tsp. dried thyme.

DIRECTIONS

1. Place a large nonstick frying pan over high heat and add 1 teaspoon of olive oil. When the oil is hot, add the pork chops and reduce the heat to medium. Sear the chops for 3 minutes on one side, flip, and sear the other side for 3 minutes, 6 minutes total. Transfer the chops to a plate and set aside.

2. In the same pan, add the remaining 1 teaspoon of olive oil. Add the apples and onion. Cook for 5 minutes or until tender, stirring frequently to prevent burning.

3. While the apples and onion cook, mix together the broth and Dijon mustard in a small bowl.

4. Add the sage and thyme to the pan and stir to coat the onion and

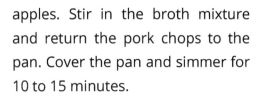

apples. Stir in the broth mixture and return the pork chops to the pan. Cover the pan and simmer for 10 to 15 minutes.

5. Let pork chops rest for 2 minutes before cutting.

NUTRITION (per serving):

Calories: 234 kcal | Fats: 11g | Carbs: 13g | Protein: 20g.

LAMB KEBABS WITH CUCUMBER DIPPING SAUCE

10 min

25 min

Beef & Pork Mains

6 Servings

INGREDIENTS

- 1 medium onion, diced
- 3 garlic cloves, minced
- Olive oil
- 1 tsp. ground cumin
- 2 tsp. fresh oregano leaves (or 1 teaspoon dried oregano)
- ¼ tsp. crushed red pepper or cayenne pepper
- 1 lb. ground lamb
- ½ cup chopped flat leaf parsley
- 1 lemon zest and

DIRECTIONS

1. Sauté the onion and 1 teaspoon of the minced garlic in 1 tablespoon olive oil over medium high heat in a small skillet until tender.

2. Add 1 teaspoon cumin, oregano, red pepper flakes and cook, stirring, for another minute - set aside to cool slightly.

3. Combine the lamb in a large mixing bowl with the onion mixture, chopped parsley and lemon zest along with 1 tablespoon olive oil, 1 teaspoon salt and 1/2 teaspoon black pepper.

4. Divide the mixture into pieces the size of golf balls and flatten two of them into a thick patty around a bamboo skewer - arrange on a platter, cover and chill for about 10

juice

- Sea salt
- Freshly ground black pepper
- ½ cup plain Greek yogurt, not fat free, use real yogurt
- ¼ cup diced cucumber
- ½ small jalapeño, stem and seeds removed.

minutes to firm. This makes 6 skewers.

5. Meanwhile, make the dressing by combining the yogurt, cucumber, remaining 1/2 teaspoon minced garlic, 1 tablespoon of the lemon juice, 1/2 teaspoon cumin, jalapeño, 1/2 teaspoon salt, 1/4 teaspoon black pepper in the blender until smooth. pour into small bowl and set aside. You can also combine in a bowl for a salsa style creamy sauce.

6. Preheat grill or grill pan and cook the lamb kebabs for 5 to 6 minutes, turning halfway through so that both sides are well browned. I grill slices of onion and sweet pepper alongside the lamb.

7. Serve warm with the dressing on the side. These are delicious.

NUTRITION (per serving):

Calories: 148 kcal | Fats: 8.7g | Carbs: 4.3g | Protein: 13g.

BELL PEPPER NACHOS

 10 min   20 min   Beef & Pork Mains   4 Servings

INGREDIENTS

- 1 lb. lean ground beef (93%)
- ⅓ cup salsa
- 2 tbsp. Taco Seasoning
- Nonstick cooking spray
- 20 to 25 mini bell peppers, halved lengthwise, trimmed, and seeded
- 1 cup Mexican cheese, shredded.

DIRECTIONS

1. Preheat the oven to 400°F.

2. In a large skillet over medium heat, brown the meat until no longer pink, breaking it up as it cooks, 7 to 10 minutes. Drain the meat and stir in the salsa and taco seasoning. Simmer for 3 to 5 minutes, until the liquid has cooked down.

3. Spray a large baking sheet with cooking spray and arrange the peppers on the sheet cut side up.

4. Fill the peppers with the beef, and sprinkle with the cheese.

5. Bake until the cheese is melted, about 5 minutes, and serve immediately

NUTRITION (per serving):

Calories: 348 kcal | Fats: 17g | Carbs: 15g | Protein: 31g.

DESSERT
RECIPES

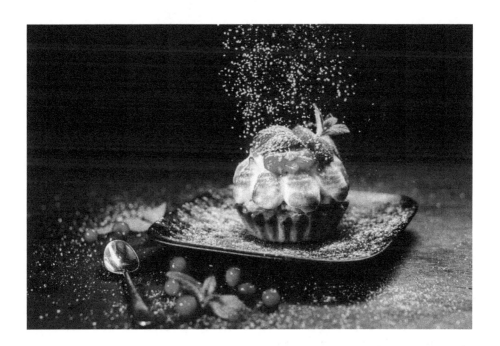

PUMPKIN PIE SPICED YOGURT

15 min	0 min	Desserts	2 Servings

INGREDIENTS

- 2 cup low-fat plain yogurt
- ½ cup pumpkin puree
- ¼ tsp. cinnamon
- ¼ tsp. pumpkin pie spice
- ¼ cup chopped walnuts
- 1 tbsp. honey.

DIRECTIONS

1. Combine spices with the pumpkin puree in a medium bowl and stir.

1. Stir in yogurt, divide into 2 serving glasses. Top with honey and walnuts. Serve and enjoy!

NUTRITION (per serving):

Calories: 207 kcal | Fats: 7g | Carbs: 22g | Protein: 6g.

TROPICAL DREAMS PUDDING

10 min

0 min

Desserts

4 Servings

INGREDIENTS

- 1 package sugar-free fat-free banana instant pudding mix
- 2 cups cold skim milk
- 4 scoops tropical fruit-flavored low-carb whey protein isolate powder.

DIRECTIONS

1. In a medium bowl, beat pudding mix, milk, and protein powder with an electric hand mixer until thoroughly blended and slightly thickened, about 2 minutes.

2. Pour pudding into 4 small bowls and refrigerate until set, about 5 minutes.

3. Serve immediately or cover and refrigerate for up to 2 days. Enjoy!

NUTRITION (per serving):

Calories:125 kcal | Fats: 10g | Carbs: 12g | Protein: 7g.

NO BAKE STRAWBERRY CHEESECAKE

2 h 20 min

0 min

Desserts

6-8 Servings

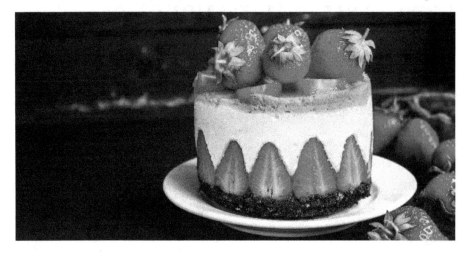

INGREDIENTS

- 8 oz. low- fat cream cheese, softened - do not use fat free
- ½ cup Stevia
- ½ cup sugar free strawberry preserves
- 1 (6-oz.) cup 2% Greek yogurt

DIRECTIONS

1. For cookie crumb crust: pulse 2/3 package oatmeal cookies with 1 tablespoon melted butter in food processor and press into pie plate or springform bottom.

2. Beat the cream cheese and Stevia, using an electric mixer, until fluffy.

3. Add the preserves, yogurt and vanilla; beat until just combined.

- 1 tsp. vanilla extract
- 2 cups Cool Whip, thawed
- ¼ cup fresh strawberries, hulled and diced
- 5-6 strawberries to slice and decorate top of pie
- 2/3 package oatmeal cookies
- 1 tbsp. melted butter.

4. Fold in the whipped topping and chopped strawberries.

5. Pile the filling into crust, smooth and either chill or freeze.

6. Remove from freezer about 20 minutes before serving to soften.

7. Arrange berry slices to decorate pie.

NUTRITION (per serving):

Calories: 120 kcal | Fats: 2.1g | Carbs: 15.5g | Protein: 4.6g.

NO SUGAR ADDED CARROT CAKE

15 min

35 min

Desserts

6-8 Servings

The cake is super moist, delicious and completely 'no added sugar' as its very lightly sweetened with stevia. It does have calories and carbs, so have a small slice.

INGREDIENTS

- ¾ cup almond flour
- ¾ cup all-purpose flour
- 1½ tsp. baking powder
- ½ tsp. salt
- 1 tsp. ground cinnamon
- ½ tsp. ground cardamom
- ½ cup Stevia
- 3 large eggs
- ½ cup plain yogurt or sour cream,

DIRECTIONS

1. Preheat oven to 350°F.

2. Spray an 8-inch round cake pan with vegetable cooking spray and line with a round of parchment or waxed paper.

3. Blend the almond flour, flour, baking powder, salt, cinnamon and cardamom in a medium bowl and set aside.

4. Whisk the Stevia, eggs, yogurt, vanilla and butter in a large bowl until creamy; add the dry ingredients and mix until just blended. Fold in the carrots.

5. Pour into prepared pan and bake

reduced fat

- 1 tsp. vanilla
- 4 tbsp. butter, melted
- 3 medium carrots, grated

FROSTING INGREDIENTS

- 4 oz. Philadelphia light cream cheese (not fat free)
- 1 cup heavy cream or whipping cream
- 1 tbsp. Jello Sugar Free Instant Vanilla Pudding powder
- ¼ cup finely chopped walnuts.

30 to 35 minutes until toothpick inserted near center comes out clean. Turn out onto cooling rack and peel off paper.

6. If making the topping: whip cream cheese until fluffy, add cream and pudding powder and beat until smooth and creamy.

7. When cake is completely cooled, scrape frosting onto center of layer, spread to edges and level.

8. Sprinkle with the walnuts.

9. Chill until serving.

NUTRITION (per serving):

Calories: 210.7 kcal | Fats: 8.9g | Carbs: 24.7g | Protein: 5.6g.

CPSIA information can be obtained
at www.ICGtesting.com
Printed in the USA
BVHW091928060721
611238BV00009B/159